YOUTHFUL IMAGINATION

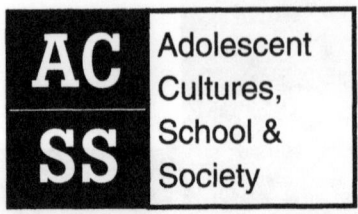

Joseph L. DeVitis & Linda Irwin-DeVitis
GENERAL EDITORS

Vol. 34

PETER LANG
New York • Washington, D.C./Baltimore • Bern
Frankfurt am Main • Berlin • Brussels • Vienna • Oxford

Georgina Tsolidis

YOUTHFUL IMAGINATION

Schooling, Subcultures, and Social Justice

PETER LANG
New York • Washington, D.C./Baltimore • Bern
Frankfurt am Main • Berlin • Brussels • Vienna • Oxford

Library of Congress Cataloging-in-Publication Data
Tsolidis, Georgina.
Youthful imagination: schooling, subcultures, and social justice / Georgina Tsolidis.
p. cm. — (Adolescent cultures, school and society; v. 34)
Includes bibliographical references and index.
1. Students—Australia—Victoria—Social conditions. 2. Student aspirations—
Australia—Victoria. 3. Subculture—Australia—Victoria. 4. Social justice—Australia—
Victoria. I. Title. II. Series: Adolescent cultures, school & society; v.34.
LC206.A8T78   306.43'209945—dc22   2006013215
ISBN 0-8204-6834-7
ISSN 1091-1464

Bibliographic information published by **Die Deutsche Bibliothek**.
Die Deutsche Bibliothek lists this publication in the "Deutsche
Nationalbibliografie"; detailed bibliographic data is available
on the Internet at http://dnb.ddb.de/.

Cover design by Zo Gay, Damage Design

© 2006 Peter Lang Publishing, Inc., New York
29 Broadway, New York, NY 10006
www.peterlang.com

All rights reserved.
Reprint or reproduction, even partially, in all forms such as microfilm,
xerography, microfiche, microcard, and offset strictly prohibited.

For Eirene and Alexis, who in different ways, have taught me a great deal about education.

Table of Contents

Acknowledgments xi

Chapter 1
Recalling Public Space 1
    Choosing Risky Identifications 5
    The Significance of Culture 6

Chapter 2
Refusing Choice as a Way of Working 9
    On Doing Ethnography in Schools 12
    Ethical Research 15
    Told and Untold Stories 15
    Where I Want the Story to Go 17

Chapter 3
The Blue or the Red Pill? 20
    Imagining that which Is Not Yet 25
    Forcing Ourselves to Face Utopia 27
    The Matrix, the Real and the Imaginary 28

Chapter 4
Coveting a Culture of Success 32
    The Fables of Tables 37
    Zoning In — The Politics of Entry 40
    Loving and Hating the Culture of Success 44
    The Cost of Community and Its Imagined Style 46
    The Loud Silence of Class 47
    Mining the Migrant Mentality 49
    Is Anything Really Priceless? 52

Chapter 5
Strategic Identities —
Pathways to Imagined Futures 55
    Seeping and Silent Cultures 64

Chapter 6
Being in 'Geek Kingdom' 68
    Jocks and Blondes 72
    Homophobic Bullying 76
    Silenced Cultures 79
    Wogs — 'It's Like a Sovereign State' 83
    In-Between Spaces 86

Chapter 7
Choosing To Perform —
'Wogs' and 'Blondes' 90

Chapter 8
'... Music Doesn't Really Cut It' —
When Music Is and Isn't Your Life 107
    Being Middling 114

Chapter 9
Synthesising Selves 123

Chapter 10
Being Mercenary —
The Politics of Performance 140
- The Everyday Experience According to Nerds 143
- Supporting Good Results 146
- Standard Measures 148
- Performing Disengagement...............149
- Managing Performance 150
- Performing Below Par 153
- School Ethos................154
- Disciplining Performance 158

Chapter 11
Disciplining for Reputation 164
- Discipline — The Dark Side of Schooling.............166
- Discipline for Learning 168
- On Being a 'Good' School.................173

Chapter 12
Imagined Futures —
Passion or Passionate Pragmatics?................179
- Fiddling with Success 181
- Focused on Being Middling................184
- Marrying Millionaires and Buying Lottery Tickets 185
- Imagined Futures 188

Chapter 13
Identity as Academic Liability 191

Bibliography 199

Index 205

Acknowledgments

Joseph DeVitis and Linda Irwin-DeVitis for providing me with the opportunity to be part of this book series.

Ian Dobson who worked with patience and good humour on many tables and graphs, some of which appear in Chapter 4.

Lawrie Angus who read the manuscript in record time, when it least suited him to do so, and provided insightful comments and invaluable feedback.

Eirene Tsolidis-Noyce, Stella Coram, Gerald Burke, Damon Anderson, Vikki Pollard, and Zo Gay who between them provided transcriptions, research assistance, statistics, 'must-have' references, indexes and art work, and most significantly, support, insights, and creative energy.

Johanna Wyn and her colleagues at the Australian Youth Research Centre for their hospitality during a recent sabbatical.

Most of all, the students, staff, and parents of Leafy Suburbs College, who allowed me into their lives.

Chapter 1

Recalling Public Space

The group of parents and students started to congregate outside the school hall. It was a night late in the academic year when student achievements would be celebrated. This was the case, particularly for the Year 12 students whose final school results were now known. As parents and students settled into their seats, a school string ensemble began to play. The neatly printed program offered the names of these performers, the schedule for the evening, and the names of students whose achievements we were there to celebrate. A vast number of these names bore witness to Australia's long history of migration.

Leafy Suburbs College is situated in the belt of suburbs that grew rapidly in order to accommodate the postwar baby boom. In comparison to the many nearby private schools, the buildings are not spectacular; standard government issue. One of several types of school buildings that dots the Victorian landscape — each school's architecture a telltale sign of its vintage. However, this school sports a few additional touches that provide an air of something more. A rose garden, a school facade with a little more flourish than most, a specially landscaped courtyard, and a school hall. Such additions represent countless fund-raising activities and much lobbying by school community and staff.

The stage is adorned with a huge pedestal and flower arrangement. The lectern is set up with a microphone and the uncomfortable seating is divided by a roped-off section for dignitaries whose titles are displayed on the back of the seats — School Principal, President of the School Council, invited members of the school community, and the evening's guest speaker. There is a feel to the event that all is not what it aspires to be. There is a little too much draft in the hall. The lack of floor covering exaggerates the 'echoey' feel of the place. The coffee is served in polystyrene cups and most parents look as though they need to be somewhere else getting ready for another hectic day at work. The Year 12 students sit together and project an en-masse look of 'Do we have to be here?' This is their last hoorah for the school. Genuine animation seems only to occur when there are exchanges with favourite teachers. So despite the flowers and the sheer delight on the teachers' faces, there is a sense of going through the motions of some other time and place; a sense that this event is proof of the teachers' enthusiasm for their work, students, and school.

Tonight's Speech Night is not an open event. With the exception of the Year 12 students, others are here by strict invitation. Students from lower year-levels who have excelled will have their names called out and they will march onto the stage and be handed an award. These are for academic, musical, or sporting excellence. After this, the Deputy Principal for the Senior School calls out a seemingly endless list of names and as she does, each student moves on to the stage. The names are not called out in alphabetical order. Instead scores above a certain grade provide the rationale for the sequence. 'The following students received scores above 80.' This sequence culminates with the Dux of the School who received a score of 99.5. She was also praised for her musical, sporting, and leadership activities. Students who received a score less than 80 remain in their seats.

I have taken a seat next to a moist-eyed grandmother who spoke heavily accented English. Later in the evening her daughter holds her gently by the elbow and points to where the child they have in common stands on the stage. There is a type of sentimentality in the hall; a sense that the community has the school in common and through it, share an interest in each other's children. Each award winner has contributed to the culture of the school by showing respect for achievement. And this is something that benefits all the students. 'School ethos' was the term the Principal had used in an informal conversation with me about what he thought makes the school special.

The long list of names read out at this Speech Night bears witness to what makes Leafy Suburbs College special. It is a school that gets its students over the line. This was a point made several times during the evening's formalities. Yet it is a school where students come from various ethnic backgrounds, with a significant number not born in Australia. The school is in a middle-class area, but includes a population that qualifies for government maintenance allowances. Indeed, some would argue that the popularity of the school has served to increase the value of surrounding properties and propel the suburb into a higher socioeconomic classification. The school is valuable because its students achieve Year 12 scores that provide them with entry into Victoria's most elite universities. Commonly this right of entry is reserved for those students who have attended elite independent and Catholic schools.

In a primary school a few kilometres away from Leafy Suburbs College a similar scene plays out. Another 'echoey' hall dressed up for the occasion. In this instance, all exiting Year 6 students are being awarded for their achievements. At the end of the evening each student stands and a short biography is read out. These culminate with the name of the secondary school the student will attend the following year. This primary school is in an inner-city area that has recently become part of the gentrification process sweeping such Melbourne suburbs. These suburbs had been working-class with large percentages of immigrants making them their own. Increasing property values reflect the wave of affluent residents moving in. Parents at this school have witnessed the value of houses purchased some time ago double or treble. Alternatively, they are well-heeled, new arrivals. The nature of this changing community is reflected in the selection of secondary schools. Most students will attend elite independent or Catholic schools, sometimes travelling across Melbourne in order to do so. Others will attend neighbourhood Catholic schools. Only a handful of students will be attending government schools, most the nearby secondary school. Two students will travel to Leafy Suburbs College.

There is a clear pecking order reflected in these choices. Those who will attend the local secondary college are those seen as having no choice, because within this community, that school is held in low regard. In the frenzied months leading up to final secondary school selection, parents congregate at the school gates exchanging the most recent hearsay on school suitability. In this context, they will tell you that there is no discipline at the local secondary school; the students there don't come from 'families like ours'; or that the progressive teaching approaches reflect the low priority given to academic excellence. The mostly unspoken subtext of the talk at the gate is that children who will attend private schools have parents who are wealthy or parents who care enough to sacrifice their lifestyle for their children's future. There is an operating assumption that price reflects quality. There are also parents who claim they are not able to send their children to a local government school that meets their requirements. Those whose children will attend Leafy Suburbs College are understood as education-literate parents, who are in the know or who have connections. It is one of very few government schools seen to offer what private schools offer and as such cannot meet the high demand for places.

> As the public sphere packs up and walks away from poor and working-class youth, it is absolutely essential for the community to recall these spaces. Those of us who work with public schools cannot sit by and accept that schools do no more than reproduce social inequalities, though this may certainly be the case much of the time. We must engage in the creation and protection of 'counterpublics' — spaces where the adults and youth can challenge the very exclusionary practices currently existing in public institutions — practices that inscribe inequality by social class, race, gender and sexuality.
>
> (Weis and Fine 2001:499)

At the heart of this exploration is whether or not a school such as Leafy Suburbs College can function as a 'counterpublic' space — somewhere that facilitates university entry for particular groups of students. On the one hand, it is a public school, and because of this, it is most often positioned in binary opposition to private schools. Yet on the other hand, it is associated with privilege — the privilege of being able to take a tilt at the windmill of an elite university education, something very few public schools can offer their students. Unlike private schools where paying high fees will open the door to university, the process by which a student accesses a place at this school is relatively opaque. In these and other ways, Leafy Suburbs College is constituted as an ambivalent location. Here, there is an interest to read this ambivalence through the experiences of the young people who are positioned within it. As the title suggests, a major interest is in social justice, an advocacy of the need to reclaim public schools as part of a social justice agenda. It has been argued that public schools can function as the front line in the battle for social justice (Nieto 2005). However, this argument is coupled with the understanding that public schools are not in themselves undifferentiated places. Within this category exist a range of differences with the potential to delimit student life choices. I have chosen to anchor this exploration to academic success, understood in relation to the scores that determine university eligibility. However, in order to resist being totally driven by normative understandings of academic success, I have also considered how students imagine their futures and understand their experience of schooling in relation to these futures. How are youthful imaginations facilitated and restricted by school structures intended to facilitate academic success?

Teese and Polesel comment that as patterns of inequality linger;

> reformers, despairing of more overt signs of progress, have abandoned the macro-sociology of education, with its ever-mounting evidence of inertia, to embrace the micro-sociology of schools. For the great diversity of schools found in any one system invites the argument that part at least of the problems of low achievement, low motivation, and early leaving lies with the power of schools themselves to fix.
>
> (Teese and Polesel 2003:185)

Whilst I am drawn to the microsociology of schooling, I do not believe that school effectiveness can dislodge the factors that contribute to the stability of the hierarchy that characterises educational achievement. Because of this, I have attempted to mediate the macrosociology of education and the microsociology of schools by considering what happens at the school level in the context of the geographies of students' educational achievements.

In an uncharacteristic flurry of optimism, I decided to look for a 'good news' story related to educational success and work backward in order to explore issues related to schooling and social justice. Leafy Suburbs College is in the Australian state of Victoria. It is a government school with a student population that is marked by difference. Whilst situated in a middle-class area, students nonetheless come from varied socioeconomic backgrounds. The school is coeducational. Many students were born outside Australia in a variety of countries and those born in Australia come from a wide range of ethnic backgrounds. Relative to other government schools, many of its students enter prestigious universities. What can the microdynamics of such a school culture tell us that may contribute to an understanding of how difference works in relation to uncomplicated definitions of success? The emphasis here is on the culture of the school as this is shaped and mediated by students rather than school culture as an ethos linked to effectiveness (McGaw, Banks, and Piper 1991; Rowe 2000). The aim is to understand student experiences of schooling and how these rub up against, colour and mediate the culture of a school that could be described as effective.

In Australia, as in many other countries, schooling and university entry is increasingly understood in relation to education markets. Much attention has been given to the relative effectiveness of private or independent schools relative to state, public, or government schools in debates about university access (Marginson 1997; Caldwell and Roskam 2002; Teese and Polesel 2003; Teese 2000). Within such debates, choice is increasingly significant. What is the basis for choice and what are its implications for individuals, communities, and society? Because Leafy Suburbs College is a government school, it is not free to charge fees of its own making nor determine, in straightforward ways, which students enter and leave. It has to function in a 'market way' but by stealth. I believe that this situation throws up in particularly stark relief the pressures and contradictions related to schooling more generally. My interest is to examine how students at this school experience the pressures and contradictions thrown up by its status.

Choice is a significant factor when education position is distributed within a market. Ball et al. argue that while a student's choice of school is pragmatic, it is also heavily imbued with the nonrational and cultural, particularly for those without a history of participation in higher education. With particular reference to the working-class and ethnic minorities, they argue that entry to elite universities needs to be understood as 'the outcome of several stages of decision-making in which choices and constraints or barriers inter-weave' (Ball et al. 2002:67). For these groups, such choice and the risk implied is pegged to becoming something different, unlike for the middle-class, where anxiety relates to 'down classing'.

Choosing Risky Identifications

The choice and risk of becoming something else is implied in the debates about schooling and social justice. In this context, identity becomes critical. What are the different identities students want to take on? And what are the identities they reject on the way to becoming something they are not already? The choice and risk implied in becoming something else is linked to social mobility expressed in class terms, but it is also linked to the 'liquidification' Bauman considers imperative to globalisation. In the context of a globalised world and its resultant cultural fluidity, he argues that 'durable identity is no more an asset; increasingly and evermore evidently, it becomes a liability. *The hub of postmodern life strategy is not making identity stand — but the avoidance of being fixed'* (Bauman 1997:89, original emphasis). Given the cultural imperatives of globalisation, becoming something different involves not only the choice, possibility, and risk of transferring between classes. It also involves the endless process of becoming, implied in Bauman's argument about the postmodern investment in nondurable identities.

In this book, Bauman's proposition is explored in juxtaposition to the sometimes strident self-identification of young people with particular youth subcultures. Of specific interest is the relationship between such subcultures and educational achievement. I am also interested in exploring the proposition provided by Eagleton (2000) that culture is not inherently political. Instead, it becomes so only if it is caught up within dynamics of domination and resistance. There are indications that ethnicity forms a particularly significant element in the politics of youth identity and the dynamics of domination and resistance as these are played out in the context of schooling. Complex relations exist between different groups of students, between each group and the teachers, and within each group in relation to factors such as gender, class, and migrancy.

Debates about social justice and education have become increasingly complex due to marketisation and the various interpretations given to increased participation by groups, such as women and girls and those from ethnic minorities, that historically have had lower rates of participation (Yates and Leder 1996; Birrell, Rapson, Dobson and Smith 2002; Collins, Kenway, and McCleod 2000). Against a backdrop of backlash politics against feminism and multiculturalism, the latter most pronounced in relation to anti-Muslim sentiments (Poynting 2002), it has become increasingly difficult to discuss students' everyday experiences of harassment. Such factors make it imperative for educationists to understand how students imagine their identities and cultural futures as these are mediated by school-based dynamics related to both social circumstance and choice.

The Significance of Culture

A long-term, ethnographic study of Leafy Suburbs College is the basis for this discussion of schooling, social justice, and how young people imagine their futures. A particular emphasis is given to student identities and how these intersect with their imagined futures. This exploration has three conceptual anchors: a straightforward link between educational success and higher education, particularly elite universities; the belief that socioeconomic status does not, on its own, unravel the complicated relationships between schools, students, and universities; and the belief that culture is central to ways of understanding the issues under consideration. Culture is understood as an ongoing process that is about meaning making (Clifford 1986; Fuchs 2001). I would like to explore both the role of the dominant culture of the school in hegemonic meaning making, and in relation to it, the 'elusive' cultures of the students — cultures that defy our capacity as teachers, researchers, and adults to pin them down and know them (Yon 2000). I explore this sense of culture as meaning making within a particular theoretical framework that acknowledges the realities of education as a market, and in this way, I attempt to engage with culture as mediated by power. Willis (2003) reminds us that there is a need to explore culture through schools given that students are the 'foot soldiers' of modernity. He suggests that ethnographic work with school students provides a bottom-up view of the interface between school culture, taken to be mainstream adult culture, and popular youth cultures.

Leafy Suburbs College is an elite government school, and as such, occupies a particular location in the education market. My aim is to consider the complex relations through which students mediate ways of knowing and being within a school that, because of its market location, offers them an inflexible understanding of academic success and the means by which it can be achieved. The book is therefore an exploration of the 'social magic' (Butler and Bourdieu 1999) that elaborates educational success through the performance of the 'good' school, and it is also an exploration of ambivalence related to such performance. Of most interest to me are student identities as they are lived within and between the market culture of the school and their own subcultures — and the ambivalence these identities reflect. My aim is also to consider students' identifications in relation to educational success. How do students mediate their identities within the culture of the school, subcultures within it, and their imagined futures? This question has the potential to speak to social justice issues because it offers an opportunity to consider how students from diverse backgrounds come to understand and perform the role of the 'good' student. When education is a market, students from increasingly diverse backgrounds engage with what are arguably more narrow and prescribed understandings of academic success. What is the relationship between difference and sameness when this occurs?

In overall terms, this exploration is guided by the question, Is it possible to succeed without assimilating? If students from the margins do succeed, is it because they have unlearned what made them different — the few in Bourdieu (1997) terms that move outside the reproductive frameworks? Perhaps instead, success implies, almost by definition, a capacity for what Spivak (1993) describes as strategic identification. In her terms, all identifications risk essentialism, but this risk may be worth taking as a form of resistance in some contexts and at some times. She argues that strategic essentialism may have merit if it is coupled with a process that allows us to question the labels we hold dear, and in so doing, guard against the consolidation of identities as essential. Spivak argues for ongoing reflexivity so that the labels behind which we rally do not become a form of entrenched identity politics. In this sense, this study is a reflexive rallying behind the label 'public school', a label held dear in social justice discourses about education. A central argument put forward in this book is that the capacity for strategic identification is a crucial element of success for students at Leafy Suburbs College. It is a public school that performs private schooling. It has limited resources and a diverse student population. Because of this, it offers a narrow and strictly adhered to conception of the 'good student'. At the micro-level, students have to become adept at strategic identifications. Their capacity to manipulate the hegemonic discursive construction of the 'good student' will be responsive to a range of factors including their own 'elusive' cultures. They are variously equipped to work within and between the hegemonic and the 'elusive' by virtue of their embodiment, class, and culture. For some, becoming this version of the 'good student' is not possible. Other students have to forgo their particular 'elusive' culture in order to perform the 'good student'. 'Good student' can become something that defines what some students do not want to become. For a select few, however, 'good student' is reinterpreted through ironic playfulness. For these students, 'good student' is a discursive space that can be occupied in transition between the every day of schooling, made bearable by 'elusive' cultures, and imagined futures that schooling might enable.

For those of us concerned with social justice issues, public schools hold a special place. Yet a public school such as Leafy Suburbs College does not immediately reconcile itself with the view of counterpublics put forward by Weis and Fine (2001). Instead of being a space 'where the adults and youth can challenge the very exclusionary practices ... that inscribe inequality by social class, race, gender and sexuality' (Weis and Fine 2001:499), at face value, it resembles a place that reinscribes such exclusionary practices. Students, regardless of their backgrounds, are expected to perform the 'good student' understood in narrow and normative ways. Yet in Melbourne, there are very few public schools that provide students with access to elite universities. In Chapter 4 this issue will be discussed in more detail. In the next two chapters, I discuss some of the theoretical issues that inform this exploration.

Chapter 2

Refusing Choice as a Way of Working

In his paper, 'Class Struggle or Postmodernsim? Yes, please!', Zizek (2000) draws on the other Marx (Groucho) to highlight what for Zizek is a major issue for those of us concerned with reconciling 'old-fashioned' politics with new ways of theorising. Zizek concludes through the words of Marx (Groucho) that answering 'Yes please!' to the question, 'Tea or coffee?', is a 'refusal of choice'. Zizek argues that this 'refusal of choice' needs to be applied also to questions that imply a choice between 'class struggle' and postmodernism. This desire to answer 'Yes, please!' and in so doing refuse 'either/or' choices, frames my exploration of schooling, social justice, and students' imagined futures at a number of levels.

The study described here has evolved through my ongoing interest in social justice, difference, schooling, and higher education. In general terms, I am concerned to explore why some students are more successful than other students if we decide 'success' equals getting into university, particularly those universities that are understood as relatively elite. Poststructural theorisations have made many of us reluctant to 'return' to clearly class-based renditions of how the world works. Teleological meta-narratives based on class dichotomies are difficult to sustain in a theoretical climate that has provided significant critiques of such theorisations, albeit at the risk of forgoing relatively neatly imagined pathways to emancipation. Hence, my attraction to Zizek's 'refusal of choice'. Transferring this logic to my study, I am interested to understand the 'hard data' related to educational achievement, but to do so without reducing the story line to one about postcodes, zip codes, or area codes as a means of explaining educational success and its relationship to socioeconomic status. I would like to understand how the students who are encapsulated by the figures experience education. We need to answer 'Yes please!' to what Teese and Polesel (2003) refer to as the 'macrosociology of education' and the 'microsociology of schools'.

A second and related refusal of choice concerns identity and the need to understand it as both fixed and fluid. When a student enters a classroom, in their teacher's mind they are already female, male, ethnic minority, working-class, 'good' or 'bad'; in short, the teacher sees them as a potential success or failure. While this fixity of identity is marked by place, time, context, and the actors involved, nonetheless it forms part of the obstacle course that sits between a student and his or her imagined future. Moreover, this obstacle course is fundamental to the shaping of any student's imagined future. The capacity to recognise that this fixity of identity is not what it appears becomes a Catch-22. Can a student who is constructed as a failure develop the wherewithal to imagine and sustain a different self-image and, if so, how does this different image in turn reiterate and challenge normative constructions of success and failure?

Zizek comments that

> what I will become depends on the interplay between contingent social circumstances and my free choice ... The crucial point here is, again, that in certain specific social conditions (of commodity exchange and a global market economy), 'abstraction' becomes a direct feature of actual social life, the way concrete individuals behave and relate to their fate and to their social surroundings.
>
> (Zizek 2000:105)

I find the relationship described by Zizek between the abstract and the actual particularly relevant. I am keen to explore the possibility that for a government school like Leafy Suburbs College to succeed in traditional terms, it needs to offer its students a very narrow interpretation of academic culture. This representation is necessarily shaped by the harsh realities of domination and subordination. Yet there is a possibility that at such a school, contingent social forces may provide students with harsh lessons in cultural choice-making that may better enable them to develop a sense of nondurable identity (Bauman 2000). For this reason, identity is understood here as the interplay between social circumstances and free choice, that is, as both fixed and fluid.

A process of becoming characterises adolescence. It is a period of transition. Rather than consider this transition as developmental — a sequential series of steps, teleological by nature — the aim is to consider students' identity as a process that is responsive to the specificities of location; in this case, Leafy Suburbs College. Students at this school, as elsewhere, grapple with identity issues. These play out most obviously through subcultures. In their early years of secondary schooling, students are introduced to a range of student subcultures. By the end of Year 10, they need to make hard choices about which subjects best facilitate their imagined futures and their place at the school. By working within and between the subcultures and the dominant cultures of the school, they 'relate their fate to their social surroundings' (Zizek 2000:105) and in the process, create identities that facilitate their imagined futures. The aim is to explore the choices young people make about their education, their identities and their adult lives through a meaning-making framework that is premised on a refusal of choice. Of central interest here is the proposition provided by Bauman who argues that culture is paradoxical in that 'whatever serves the preservation of a pattern undermines its grip' (2000). In this sense, rather than 'an anti-randomness device' (Bauman 2000) culture is given lived meaning in relation to difference and becoming within the context of Leafy Suburbs College.

Just as students' identities are transient and responsive to situationality, so too is the identity of the author. While there are clear limitations to the argument that all text is simply autobiographical, it would be foolhardy to ignore the biographical element. In this text, I come to the task of researching and writing about young people, their schools, and their imagined futures as someone with an ongoing interest and involvement in education. I have taught in secondary schools considered disadvantaged, worked in bureaucracies with responsibility for policy related to social justice, and currently work in the faculty of education at a large university. Perhaps more than any of these responsibilities, my location as a parent of two teenage school children influences my thinking most dramatically. This brings me to another refusal of choice, between agency and structure. As we write texts on schools, there can be a tendency to forget that students have a capacity to see through our versions of their reality.

As a parent I have been involved in the processes I describe: the frenzied chatting at the school gates about school choice, the exploration of school performativity, the hearsay about school cultures, discipline, the range of subjects offered, and the types of families in attendance. We all want the best for our children regardless of how we constitute 'best'. At the end of the day, however, it was my children who made the decision about the school they wanted to attend. My daughter preempted what she thought may be my preference for single-sex schooling by announcing one day in very firm tones that she had no intention of attending a girls' secondary school. She had researched and rehearsed the arguments in favour of coeducation and this was a productive exercise for her at many levels. Similarly, she made it very clear that she had even less intention of sitting an exam for entry into a selective government school. My son, likewise, was adept with his own preemptive strategic action. My children understood that with an education-literate mother they had to be one step ahead in order to stay in control. Whilst children may not be able to select their parents, they can select their schools! My ignoring their school preference would have opened the potential of them starting secondary school with deep misgivings about my choice for their futures. Starting school with confidence and enthusiasm for your school seems an important first step for any student. Parents feature in explorations of school choice (Vincent 2001; Ball 2003; MacGuire, Ball and McCrae 2001), however, student agency can be underestimated, not only with reference to school choice but also with reference to how chosen schools are experienced and influenced by their participation.

In line with Zizek's wish to answer 'Yes please!' to both the tea of class struggle and the coffee of postmodernism, I wish to explore schooling at Leafy Suburbs College by employing seemingly contradictory epistemological frameworks. It may be possible to combine the facts and figures that presume to describe a modernist real with a postmodern scepticism that the real exists. If everything is a fiction, then the real is as unreal as anything else and therefore as valid a fiction as the word captured at a particular moment in time, text, or image. Yet it is the fables of tables that gel in the imagination of those who 'get their hands dirty' with the every day of schooling. Tables that represent scores and school league tables matter for parents selecting schools, students understanding the worth of a school, or those who attend to policy. Such facts and figures create a recognisable snapshot of what is 'out there'. My aim is to read students' experiences of schooling, which is sometimes taken as not mattering, through the snapshots provided by other texts, including those most often taken as mattering, including tables. How is a school that is established as 'good' through the fables of tables experienced by students? And how do we come to understand their experiences through the fables they tell us and how we understand these?

On Doing Ethnography in Schools

I entered the carpeted foyer of the school after having followed the semicircular concrete path past the rose garden and the sign asking all visitors to report to the general office. The busy caretaker, garden clippers in hand, smiled as I passed him. Standing in front of the glassed counter behind which several women were busy either answering phones or flicking through papers, I was struck by the immediate surroundings. A flower arrangement in front of student art work, a wooden cabinet that housed school trophies, a notice board displaying newspaper clippings related to the school and its students, and a sign directing visitors' attention to the office of the school bursars. Nearby large wooden honour boards displayed the names of school captains stencilled in gold. The corridors beyond this neat foyer were filled with the energy of young people — excited chatting, broad smiles, enthusiasm, and a sense that they were happy to be there. Each student wore the required uniform, some with an added twist but nothing too out of the ordinary. The Principal walked toward me and extended a hand in introduction. I was here to explain my work and he was ready to introduce me to his school and indicate his willingness to participate in a project that may provide insights into what was working for the school and what may need improving. Our brief conversation illustrated his deep commitment and knowledge of the school and its broader community. Students greeted him with friendly smiles and conversation. He presented as a fatherly rather than distant figure.

A year into the project I entered the school foyer and once again greeted the Principal. I had arranged to interview a new staff member that morning. It was her first year at the school and she had kindly volunteered her only free period for the day. Amidst the early morning bustle of students and staff, we hurriedly occupied a conveniently located free room. It was the formal meeting room, the window of which looked out onto the well cared for courtyard. I couldn't help but notice the exchange of glances between the Principal and the teacher. He knew what I was doing and she knew he knew. Nothing was said, when later, he apologised and entered the room where the interview was being conducted in order to deposit something in preparation for an evening meeting.

In overall terms, the study captured here could be described as ethnographic. I maintained a research relationship with the school for over two years. In this period, I conducted interviews. I scrutinised documentation related to the school. I participated in the everyday life of the school through attendance at special events and just 'milling around', which provided insights. Additionally, figures related to university admissions were analysed in order to place this school and its students in a broader context. All these methods assume a research stance and perspective on the constitution of knowledge.

Traditional anthropological understandings of ethnography assume there is a 'truth' out there to be captured by the researcher and transferred to a readership. Within education, there is a common assumption that such research will make things better — better classroom practice, better policy, or better understandings of particular groups of students or teachers' work. However, for researchers who have developed a sceptical stance about the possibility of capturing a 'truth' out there, there is persistent discussion of the complexities involved in doing ethnographic research (Britzman 1995; Stronach and MacLure 1997). The emphasis has shifted to reflexivity as a means of laying bare the researcher's situationality and the power relations implicit in the research dynamic by virtue of this location. As researchers, we need to account for the perspective implicit in our gaze and its potential to colonise those we describe (Weis and Fine 2000). Within education, where research has a strong traditional link to 'making things better', an emphasis on reflection and constructivism is being questioned because of what is seen as its limited relevance to practice. Yates (2004) argues that regardless of our aims as education researchers, we do not have the luxury of sealing off ourselves by talking only to each other. Our work is also shaped from within the field, in relation to schools and the young people whose identities schools shape. Ways of researching are always contested, and what may be satisfying to some, in one context, will be rejected by others in another context. Because of this, Yates (2004) argues that education researchers need to be mindful of how our work may be situated.

This study is situated in relation to a range of debates about school choice, school effectiveness, student subcultures, and identities and access to higher education. The primary aim is to consider students' lived experiences of a school that is located ambiguously. Leafy Suburbs College is a government school but it is also seen as a 'pretend private' school. It is a school where students are under enormous pressure to gain the academic results that make this school one of the best performing in this school sector. I expect that those interested in social justice issues will gain insights from these student experiences. On occasions, I have spoken about this project at forums where teachers are present. There is an immediate interest in how the school gets its excellent results. There is interest to find out what happens at the school that enables it to be effective, and how this can be emulated at other government schools seeking better results for their students. Sometimes academics listening will be unsympathetic toward the school. Their interest turns to selection by stealth — the preemptive means by which Leafy Suburbs College includes and excludes the students most and least likely to achieve good results. Various interests reflect different professional and personal circumstances. Nonetheless, there is always interest in the words of students. As teachers or researchers, we find young people, their words, and experiences beguiling. It is the stuff of our profession. The study reported on here strives to be 'student-centric' and invites reflection on the possibility of interpreting student experiences as both a valid form of research and also a form of ventriloquism — a means whereby researchers talk through the mouths of those with whom they speak.

This study could be described as 'new ethnography' (Saukko 2003). Implicit in the approach are a range of tensions. There is an aim to acknowledge the validity of the personal, including the emotional side of lived experience. I aim to bring into light perspectives or experiences that may not be constituted through the dominant discourses and to understand that the researcher's capacity to do this is limited by the perspective implicit in their situationality and their authorial power. Various modes of writing and presenting material are used in an attempt to evoke lived experience and its representation. However, I also acknowledge that lived experience is situated within wider social processes and structures that need to be scrutinised. 'New ethnography' represents a balancing act 'of being true to the lived and being aware of the commitments and limits of its "truth"' (Saukko 2003:56).

Ethical Research

As a researcher I did not want to betray the trust the school placed in me when they opened their doors to scrutiny. When education is a market, it is not remarkable that school communities can be simultaneously reluctant to say no to research (appearing unwelcoming of scrutiny) and yes to research (loosing control of the image manufacturing increasingly at the heart of schooling). In such circumstances the ethics of research become intensely complex, particularly when there is prodding and poking behind the official storylines through the words of students, teachers, and parents. Schools become networked communities through neighbourhood, professional, and academic associations. For the researcher this creates an ethical intensity that is born of contradictory desires. There is the desire to respect the work done by school staff, whose priority is the interests of students and their school. The desire not to jeopardise students' futures through disturbing what is the fragile balancing act of school reputation. Yet there is also the desire to maintain the integrity of research as a process that allows the familiar to become unfamiliar. 'Researcher' can be understood as a privileged location that affords the opportunity for someone on the outside to say things on behalf of those on the inside who may have misgivings about what is constituted as the lived experience of their everyday through official school discourses. For many people interviewed for this study, speaking to the researcher was itself a dangerous investment. It provided them with an opportunity to make statements they felt transgressed the official school discourses to someone they thought had the right reasons for listening. Because of this trust, the researcher has the responsibility to weigh up the cost and benefit of making information public. A key element in making ethnography ethical is confidentiality. Confidentiality produces a paradox for the researcher — simultaneously providing as much information as possible and keeping aspects of this information opaque. There are many intended silences in this text, premised on the need to keep the school and individuals within it unidentifiable.

Told and Untold Stories

Leafy Suburbs College was chosen on the basis of figures related to university entry. It is one of a handful of government schools in urban Melbourne where students gain scores high enough to enter prestigious universities. Of these schools, a single-sex girls' school and single-sex boys' school, are selective entry schools that admit students at Year 9 on the basis of examination. A criterion for selecting the case study school was diversity of student population. This eliminated the select-entry schools from consideration and made Leafy Suburbs College an appropriate choice. Interviews with students were arranged through key members of staff and using snowball techniques whereby students recommended other students and teachers to be approached. The aim was to select student interviewees who were understood to be members of particular subcultures. Students were interviewed individually, in pairs, or groups on the basis of their nominated friendships. Students interviewed were also observed in a variety of contexts. Staff, parents, and former students were selected through the same means, although in the case of teachers, specific approaches were made in order to include a mix of relatively junior and senior members of staff. Interviews with students and teachers were conducted at the school. Nonteaching staff, parents, and former students were interviewed in homes.

In order to conduct school-based research, the researcher needs to clear university ethics procedures, needs the permission of the school principal, the permission of the bureaucracy which has its own ethics clearance procedures, the permission of the regional director, the permission of interviewees and, in the case of students under 18 years, their parents' permission. There are also informal processes that limit the researcher's ability to research. The research reported here was coloured by what could be achieved in the in-between spaces of the very structured processes of running a large school. Snatching interviewees between classes, in spare periods, between bells and sirens. Finding rooms to sit in and wait while students paraded past, noticed me, remembered, and ran to call friends. This process had its limitations and strengths. Because it did not rely on official school processes such as year-level coordinators selecting and calling students out of class, it had an informal, grassroot feel that I believe students found more natural. Of course, this reliance on word of mouth meant that many subgroups of students did not participate in the study. There were groups that were talked about by interviewees but not interviewed. During the course of this research, it became more or less difficult to conduct interviews with various groups of students. The exercise of naming individuals as members of subgroups was delicate. Initial contact was based on hearsay. Students were also asked to invite their friends to the interviews. I assumed that students would nominate like-minded friends and in so doing, constitute interview groups that represented particular subcultures. One of the insights gained through this process relates to the fact that friendship groups may not strictly overlap with student subcultures.

Perhaps it is those with whom you cannot speak who have the most interesting stories. Here I wish to acknowledge the silences — the stories I could not get that I knew were worth listening to and telling. In my experience in working with Leafy Suburbs College, the most interesting silences related to the newly arrived students, those described by other students as the 'Asians' and the 'Russians'. These were the quiet students, who did their work, even at lunch times. These students were not part of the circles of students who were easy to include. Understandably, the teachers were reluctant to constitute them as a group by naming them 'Russians' or 'Asians' and withdrawing them from classes so that they could be presented to the researcher for scrutiny. Previous research experience had also taught me that the very act of naming students 'Chinese', 'British' or 'South African' constitutes for them an identity and erases difference within and between such categories. Even if students are given the choice of which category to belong to, complexity is erased (Tsolidis 2001). The second significant silence was the students who left the school at the end of Year 9 or 10. These students were constructed as not good enough, as not academic, or as better off somewhere else — learning a trade, working in service industries, or attending schools with less imposing academic standards. Informal conversations with a range of such students provided insights that inform what is written here, as do descriptions of them offered by their peers and teachers. However, none was willing to be interviewed, including one young man who agreed and then managed to 'evade' me for two years. The third silence relates to the students who never made it into Leafy Suburbs College despite their and their parents' best efforts. After a while I stopped trying to interview such people and came to recognise their nice ways of saying no, which sometimes including saying yes initially. It seems more worthwhile to try to understand silence than to try to interpret stories told through gritted teeth by reluctant interviewees. Those who were interviewed shape this research and as in all research, they have provided a fragmented and partial picture. This picture is influenced by the researcher and her priorities. It also reflects how participants understood the researcher and her priorities and responded to them through the interviews and informal discussions.

Where I Want the Story to Go

Spivak (1993) makes the point that we should not underestimate the readers' capacity to take our texts to places we had not intended them to go. Research relies on readers' capacities to interpret what is written through their own experiences, and their understanding of the writer and her intentions. As authors, we can only speak in open ways about what we see ourselves doing and why we have chosen to do things in particular ways as a means of providing readers with insights into where we would like our words to go. I wish to make clear where I would like this story to go so that the reader can account for this when he or she takes it to his or her own preferred destination.

I hope to render visible some of the lived experiences within Leafy Suburbs College, an elite government school, and situate these experiences in relation to the school's broader social context. I believe that an examination of an elite government school speaks to social justice issues. Compared to many government schools, Leafy Suburbs College is well resourced. The neighbourhood is relatively affluent and, compared to many other schools, its students are well-off in a range of ways. Yet compared to many elite independent and Catholic schools, the school, the students, and the community are not well-off. If we are to assume that elite universities and elite courses are not the sole domain of those who attend elite schools, it is left to very few government schools to contribute to the mix. I would like to explore how manufacturing a 'pretend private' school impacts on students, teachers, and parents, and how this speaks to a more equitable system of schooling.

The balancing act 'of being true to the lived and being aware of the commitments and limits of its "truth"' (Saukko 2003:56) that is implicit in new ethnography is evident in the shape of this book. A range of texts are included: discursive accounts or portraiture of school events, policy documents, and interview material. I do not present my observations and interview material as a form of naive realism reminiscent of traditional ethnography. Instead, I present this material as a collage of insights that allows the reader to make the most of the stories I tell and my intentions in telling them — an attempt at 'making the familiar strange rather than the strange familiar' (Van Maanen 1995:20). These are my descriptions of my experiences of participating in the life of the school. They are real to the extent that they happened and I experienced them. They are unreal to the extent that anyone else immersed in the same events would experience these differently and describe them in different ways. I have included some documents produced by the school. Again, while this may tell us about how the school represents itself, I have selected what to put in and where it goes. The book tells stories overtly, but it is the covert stories that I would like to draw attention to from the outset. The collage of texts is far from innocent in terms of what is included and the ways in which the different material is juxtaposed. This is a case of 'Reader Beware'. The texts created and selected, and the way they have been positioned, reflect what I found interesting and the related complexities I am attempting to understand.

Alvesson and Skoloberg (2000) use the metaphor of the market to describe different approaches to knowledge. They argue that the domination of the financial market in the 1980s led to the dominance of ways of thinking that privileged the sign 'elusive images or chimeras which live their own ephemeras and capricious lives without being moored to any other reality than themselves' (159). The 1990s, however, were marked instead by recession and less optimism in the free market model. This in turn led to an exploration of postmodern thought as 'markocentric'. Alvesson and Skoloberg put forward an alternative to a market view of knowledge, one that works between absolutely sovereign actors and absolutely sovereign textuality. Instead they place an emphasis on dialogue, not as mediation of meaning, but as a means of creating knowledge in a discursive field. 'This does not mean a rational, perfect, noise-free communication; noise, friction, misunderstanding, irritation and "trouble" will always be there, and are indeed a precondition for the process' (159). This view of creating knowledge through noisy dialogue, a process in which neither the actors nor the dialogue are sovereign, guides this exploration of young people, their schooling, and imagined futures. There is no attempt to negotiate a meaning from the various perspectives — to compare what students said to what teachers said and how I experienced the school. Instead, I hope to elaborate students' 'irritation' with the structures of their schooling, as well as the means by which they work through their discovery that the adult world is not always rational. The text is an attempt to illustrate the noise and friction implicit in the every day of these young people's schooling. Following Alevsson and Skoloberg's argument, it is an attempt to go beyond the market as a way of knowing a school caught within market forces, through noisy communication with those who live this and those who are reading about how I experienced this school.

Chapter 3

The Blue or the Red Pill?

For many years I have had the responsibility of teaching sociology of education to students in their second year of a teaching degree. Mostly, this class is made up of young people who finished their own secondary schooling one year previously. During this subject, we explore the interrelationship between schooling and society and, in particular, the possibility of education being other than reproductive of social inequality. These are issues the students have lived but not necessarily thought about in a systematic way. After all, they have just begun making the transition from school student to teacher. Placements in a variety of schools are part of this course and for most students it is their first opportunity to experience a school other than the one they attended as school students. The placement experience becomes a very real lesson in understanding that education is far from a level playing field. Many of these university students were themselves educated in elite private schools. For some of these students, the school placement can be their first experience of visiting a public school and can reinforce a strong belief that the private system is superior. In turn, such schools become their preferred professional destination, thus completing the cycle. For those educated in government schools, their first visit to an elite independent or Catholic school can illustrate in a very real sense, the extreme resource discrepancies that exist between the various schooling systems. This realisation prompts various responses. For some, there is a strong sense of injustice (newly realised or already established and refuelled). The response to this can be wishing to right a wrong by teaching in the type of school they had attended themselves and in this way, they hope to work toward improving a system about which they have deep misgivings. For others, there is a flight response — a desire to work in a private school and enjoy, as teachers, the benefits they did not experience as school students.

In my efforts to teach to social justice issues, I draw on the film *The Matrix*. In this iconic science fiction film The Matrix is the means by which the artificial intelligence that has taken humans captive, allows the real world, desolate and unattractive, to appear attractive. The Matrix is the system that produces the fiction that all is well. Through their use of technology, a band of rebels see beyond this simulator and invite others, who also have become suspicious about the nature of their world, into the 'real' by severing themselves from The Matrix. If they choose this path, they are wrenched from The Matrix and reborn into an austere existence on board a pirate spaceship called the Nebuchadnezzar. Here, a bland gruel that forms their dietary mainstay tastes as it should. For those still attached to The Matrix, the same gruel tastes like anything they imagine themselves eating. On the Nebuchadnezzar, appetites are sustained by the struggle for liberation from a pleasant fantasy and the hope of passage into a desolate reality. The decision to leave The Matrix is triggered by Morpheas who is the leader of the rebels. In his quest to find The One — the person whose initial programming allows for the ultimate escape — Morpheas provides individuals with a choice between the desolate real and the imagined. In so doing, he warns them that if they chose to see things as they really are, there will be no turning back because they will have understood the truth. In this film, the real sullies the artistry of the imagined.

In my class The Matrix becomes a powerful metaphor for an exploration of hegemony within the system of schooling. Once you realise that meritocracy is a smokescreen for a reality that rewards something else, can you go back to a view that assumes schooling is benign? This is the choice that Neo, the hero of the film, is given by Morpheas — to take the blue pill and remain within the fantasy of The Matrix or to take the red pill and be plunged into a new, albeit harsh and uncompromising way of understanding. Many of my students choose the blue pill and in various ways accept living within The Matrix of meritocracy. For some of these students, schooling like other resources is simply distributed according to fortune (the good luck to have enough money!). Others believe that talent and hard work are rewarded. Some of those who choose to take the red pill are happy to remain trapped in the realisation that the system is not fair and become cynical, or paternalistic, toward students 'less well-off'. Some are like the Nebuchadnezzar rebel Cipher, who eventually sells out his friends. He chooses to go back to the comfort of The Matrix even though he knows that the thick juicy steak and red wine he is consuming in his imagination is really the same gruel he has been eating on the other side. Some students become like the rebels, willing to believe that social change is possible and that schooling has a central role to play in this process.

The Matrix engages with issues that have interested social theorists for many years. It explores how systems of inequality are understood, experienced, and camouflaged; how we as individuals, make decisions about our place in such system; and whether alternatives to the status quo are possible and how they are achieved. And for those of us concerned centrally with education, how do processes such as schooling engage with such debates? It is not surprising that someone like me, who grew up intellectually in the 1960s and 1970s, would find the issues with which *The Matrix* engages fascinating and familiar. Rebellion born of idealism and romantic, heroic tales of struggle for a better system were the pumping heart of the sixties and seventies (DeKoven 2004). But how do the young people who sit in my classes understand this dystopian science fiction parable? How do they understand my clumsy attempts to insert such narratives into their frames of reference? Are they willing/able to construct *The Matrix* as other than another stimuli for an assessment requirement that has to be successfully completed on terms constituted by those who grade it? Can they see the issues, it raises as relevant to their own schooling experiences or those of the students they imagine themselves teaching ? And more to the point, if they are taken by the heroic tale, is this useful for them?

The topic and the approach taken in this book are moulded by my reluctance to let go of a way of thinking that is seemingly outdated. The humanist project of imagining a better society and organising a means of achieving it has been fundamentally challenged. Yet why is it difficult for people like me to let go of what is essentially a political project born of Enlightenment thinking — the quest for a better system (of schooling) — even when we understand the Enlightenment meta-narrative as possibly one of the biggest fictions? This question and the concepts it presumes, including imagination, utopia, and ideology, are fundamental to this exploration. Perhaps this hankering for a political project is what DeKoven (2004) calls the 'persistence of utopian hope', something she argues is caught up with 'the structure of feeling of the sixties'. She concludes that

> if we understand how our current postmodern conjuncture emerged from the utopian modernity of the sixties, and still, in very different forms, carries some of its promise, we can recognise the popular, egalitarian, specific, muted, ironic, ambiguous, carefully pitched, disconnected, multiform, multigenre, cross-cut, sampled, electronic, hybrid, transnational, border-crossing, nomadic, multilingual, wavering or roaring voices, often misheard or misinterpreted, of that promise when they speak.

(DeKoven 2004:290)

DeKoven's central argument is that the sixties, which have been characterised as solidly Enlightenment or modern, were nonetheless pregnant with the postmodern. For her, postmodern possibilities are enriched through the assimilation of the sixties into the 'contemporary cultural political imaginary' (289). This is a resolution with which I am very comfortable because at a basic level it is utilitarian, allowing reflexive engagement with both the modern and postmodern.

Within teleological narratives of social development, change requires effort and also the capacity to imagine and believe in an alternative. An ability to consider that something is not only different, but better, is a necessary part of the change process. For example, you need to be able to imagine a better system of schooling in order to make efforts to alter the status quo seem worthwhile. Most commonly the possibility of standing outside what is commonly accepted as the normal or appropriate way of doing things, is linked to understandings of ideology. Within such understandings, education and specifically schooling, have been linked to processes that teach people to understand and accept the system and their place within it. The capacity to see beyond what you are taught to accept is linked to ideology and its self-fulling role. Embedded within this is the notion of false consciousness, that is, the belief that the system perpetuates itself by convincing people of its merits. In the context of schooling, for example, students come to understand their worth and their potential in relation to the grades they receive, rather than understand the grades as possibly indicative of what is wrong with the system.

Ideology is commonly associated with traditional conflict theories. In such theories, the prevalence of a particular ideology that favours dominant interests, explains why the oppressed may not come to understand their oppression and move toward changing the system. Ideology serves the same purpose as The Matrix. Dominant ways of understanding rely on teleological Enlightenment narratives linked to linear development toward a greater good. These are mediated by and on behalf of the humanist subject. For supporters of such Enlightenment narratives, these are juxtaposed to poststructural theories of difference that challenge the possibility of any form of universalism, the possibility that there is a perspective or an experience that speaks to all. Instead, poststructuralism emphasises situationality, a belief that any storyline reflects the experiences and interests of the interlocutor. In other words whose 'good' is constructed as common within narratives of social justice? Can Neo be everyone's One or is he simply The One that is spawned by Morpheas's imagination, itself situated by his experience? Is Neo The One because he comes to believe in himself the way Morpheas believes in him? Who we become reflects the faith others show in us and our ability to assimilate this into our imagined futures. This is a critical consideration for teachers concerned with social justice. Without some utopian vision, it is difficult for us to imagine different futures for those students, who we understand to be outside spaces traditionally reserved for the successful.

Poststructural perspectives that champion difference under the guise of progressivism are targeted with a particular vitriol by those committed to political projects of emancipation. 'The postmodern sign, whether financial or linguistic, is epistemologically false and ethically degenerate. Postmodernism is thus the veritable apotheosis of ideology' (Hawkes 2003:10). Some, nostalgic for 'pre-postmodern' ways of understanding, target groups such as feminists, as responsible for rupturing the coherence of the subject (Eagleton 2000). In this context, postmodernism becomes the ideology of global capitalism and those who support it are like Cipher, willing to betray their progressive allies for the comfort of living within the chimera created by The Matrix. In this case, however, the chimera itself is the belief that Enlightenment meta-narratives no longer hold explanatory power. Hawkes continues:

> Once capitalism has achieved a certain level of prosperity for practically all its denizens, the charms of the commodity may come to seem preferable to the arduous and dangerous quest for revolution. The fact that one's consciousness is reified, that one sees only appearances and representations rather than the things-in-themselves, may come to seem rather unimportant ... The task of philosophy from this point on is the critical negation of this virtually universal false consciousness.
>
> (Hawkes 2003:112)

Again, Zizek (2000) offers us refusal of choice as a way forward. Through the example of Marx (Groucho), he asks us to answer 'Yes Please!' to both the tea of 'old-fashioned' politics and the coffee of new ways of theorising ideology. He suggests that we can refuse to choose between accepting and rejecting ideology. On the one hand, the acceptance of ideology as the gap between the imagined and the real assumes that a real is possible. Zizek suggests that this is not a useful construction given his understanding that reality is mediated by ideology. On the other hand, he describes as slick, the postmodern response to this paradox, which is to reject the possibility of reality altogether. Instead, he argues,

> although no clear line of demarcation separates ideology from reality, although ideology is already at work in everything we experience as 'reality' we none the less maintain the tension that keeps the critique of ideology alive ... ideology is not all; it is possible to assume a place that enables us to maintain a distance from it, *but this place from which one can denounce ideology must remain empty, it cannot be occupied by any positively determined reality* — the moment we yield to this temptation, we are back in ideology.
>
> (Zizek 1994:17, original emphasis)

Going back to The Matrix, like Groucho Marx answering 'Yes please!' to both tea and coffee, can we answer 'Yes Please!' to both the red and blue pill? Can we chase the white rabbit to the Nebuchadnezzar, constructed as the empty space from which we both accept and denounce ideology as a system that explains us as duped into a condition whereby the gruel we consume is transformed into steak and wine?

Zizek identifies ideology as 'a matrix that regulates the relationship between visible and non-visible. Between imaginable and non-imaginable, as well as the changes in this relationship' (1994:1). He comments that today it seems easier for people to imagine the destruction of the planet than to imagine a fairer social system. In this way, the capacity to see beyond what is identified as already there is critical to debates about change. There is both the capacity to see what is going on behind the 'charms of the commodity' as well as the capacity to see what lies beyond the 'dangerous quest for revolution' — the capacity to imagine that which is not yet.

Imagining that which Is Not Yet

I have a deep suspicion that those of us who choose to teach are drawn to the possibility of making a difference. We are prone to constructing better places — classrooms, schools, societies — through engagements with learning. This vision is itself a grand Enlightenment trope! Yet for many, this is what gives our work meaning. The link between education and a capacity to make a difference is strong. This is evidenced by my everyday reality of teaching within undergraduate education courses. In these courses, I ask students to reflect on the reasons they have chosen a future in teaching. These neophytes are confident in nominating as a major reason for selecting teaching as a profession the desire to make a difference. Students comment that their aim is to make the world a better place by influencing young people. The following comments illustrate this.

> Like instead of just going to a business and making money for some dude that you don't even know, you actually are like doing something and it's sort of more productive in people's lives. (Ryan)

> I'm really looking forward to providing the kids with some sort of direction in life. How that works out I don't know. (Daniel)

> In secondary [schools] it's a lot more, and you can see the changes that are made ... for me I need to see that I'm sort of making a difference. (Conrad)

The idealism and altruism of these prospective teachers is characteristic of the teaching profession. An Australian Commonwealth report (Commonwealth of Australia, 1998), for example, indicated that many teachers considered acting as change agents part of their professionalism and felt that this was inadequately acknowledged and appreciated. Along similar lines, women in the profession felt that the relatively low remuneration and conditions of the profession were offset to a certain extent by the intrinsic worth of the profession as one that made a difference (Milligan 1994). This capacity to imagine a better society and believe that as teachers we can contribute to its realisation is a characteristic of teaching and one increasingly under threat (O'Brien and Schillaci 2002).

A vision of making a difference through education can become lost between the postmodern critique of it as a quaint Enlightenment narrative and the menacing vision of education as simply a private commodity linked to market models. Yet there are those who argue that it is increasingly important to hang on to a view that constructs education as significant for social change. Jacques Delors as Chairman of the Commission responsible for the inquiry into education for the twenty-first century provides a critical example of this position. In the report, *Learning: The Treasure Within* (UNESCO Publishing/The Australian National Commission for UNESCO, 1998), he titled his contribution 'Education: The Necessary Utopia'. His is an unequivocal declaration that education has an increasingly important role to play given the advent of globalisation.

He states:

> In confronting the many challenges that the future holds in store, humankind sees in education an indispensable asset in its attempt to attain the ideal of peace, freedom and social justice. As it concludes its work, the Commission affirms its belief that education has a fundamental role to play in personal and social development. The Commission does not see education as a miracle cure or a magic formula opening the door to a world in which all ideals will be attained, but as one of the principal means available to foster a deeper and more harmonious form of human development and thereby to reduce poverty, exclusion, ignorance, oppression and war.
>
> At a time when educational policies are being sharply criticised or pushed — for economic and financial reasons — down to the bottom of the agenda, the Commission wishes to share this conviction with the widest possible audience, through its analyses, discussions and recommendations.
>
> ... the Commission did its best to project its thinking on to a future dominated by globalisation, to choose those questions that everyone is asking and to lay down some guidelines that can be applied both within national contexts and on a worldwide scale.
>
> (UNESCO 1998:13–15)

Delors makes the point that he does not resile from the criticism that his recommendations are utopian. This is something he celebrates when he asks us to consider the benefits of 'imagining the best'.

The UNESCO report and Delors' declaration in favour of the utopian raise significant questions including how we understand the nature of the 'best' we imagine and who has the privilege to imagine this 'best'. The 'best' is culturally situated and manifests itself through a range of complex power relations, which are played out through significant and unequal movements between the local and global. In other words, our capacity to imagine the best, let alone attain what it is we imagine, is culturally situated and mediated by the everyday inequalities that often remain unresponsive to the ideal. Nonetheless, I find Delors' declaration an important and useful one.

We live in increasingly pragmatic cultures where idealism is denounced or at least pushed and pulled so that it can be jammed into frameworks established by the 'real'. The 'real', in turn, is construed in relation to the market. This trend of establishing a market-driven 'real' is increasingly evident in education. Delors' declaration for imagining the best, with all its attendant limitations, is important because in the context of such debates it reiterates, in unselfconscious ways, the important role education should play in contributing to the common good. It also establishes that the common good is considered within and between the local and the global.

I would like to keep alive Delors' concept of 'imagining the best' because I believe it brings significant meaning to our role as educationists. However, I also wish to acknowledge that unless we reflect on how 'best' is determined and in whose imagination it is constituted, we run the risk of promulgating yet another version of hegemonic benevolence. It is the tension between the real and the imagined, or the pragmatic and the utopian, which I believe is potentially productive. Here I am counselled by the feminist scholar Benhabib (1995) who, in reviewing the possibility of maintaining a political project and dismantling the Enlightenment subject, argues that postmodernism can represent a retreat from utopia which feminists should resist. Rather than Enlightenment utopias, including those of socialism, Benhabib links the concept of utopia to a longing 'for that which is not yet', and argues that, there is a practical-moral imperative to resist its abandonment. In the context of feminism, she argues,

> Postmodernism can teach us the theoretical and political traps of why utopias and foundational thinking can go wrong, but it should not lead to a retreat from utopia altogether.
>
> (Benhabib 1995:30)

Forcing Ourselves to Face Utopia

Raymond Williams (1980) uses a discussion of science fiction literature to consider the role of the utopian more broadly. Through science fiction, authors have been able to imagine alternative social forms. Williams explores the differences between a utopian vision, one that imagines a new set of institutions (a systematic mode), and one that is heuristic, less confident, and that targets instead a 'discourse of alternative values' (a heuristic mode). Williams argues that both modes have strengths and weaknesses. The structural mode grows out of relations that are oppressive and is premised on a strong belief that a better world is possible. However, he argues that within this model there is an emphasis on organisation and because of this, human experience can be overlooked. On the other hand, the heuristic mode grows out of 'constrained reformism' and 'can settle into isolated and in the end sentimental "desire", a mode of living with alienation' (Williams 1980:23). He argues that such utopian modes of thinking have been replaced with dystopias. These reflect the minority cultures of exiles and refugees who do not attempt collectively to change the system but instead, seek a 'hiding place, beyond both the system and the fight against the system' (Williams 1980:207). Williams uses *The Dispossessed* by Le Guin to signal the return of a different type of utopia where abundance can be achieved in non- or anti-utopian ways. This relative abundance means that within the state of affluence there is a tendency to reject from within 'by learning and imagining the condition of the excluded *others* (Williams 1980:211, original emphasis). Here, the bleak and arid landscapes become utopian because they come to symbolise the moral high ground. Unlike dystopias, these are not cynical but seek new forms of responsibility and relationships beyond those of mutuality.

Imagining utopias may provide a means of exploring schooling and social justice. As discussed above, Zizek links imagination to the matrix of ideology that controls what we can and cannot imagine. He argues that we find it easier to imagine the destruction of the planet, a dystopia, than to imagine a just social system or a new form of utopia. In his argument in support of new utopias, Williams refers to E.P. Thompson's call for an 'education of desire'. As teachers, we need to relearn this desire and explore it with our students.

The Matrix, the Real and the Imaginary

If we are to consider the education of desire — the capacity to imagine 'something that is not yet' (Benhabib 1995) as important, exploring the construction of desire seems imperative. Grosz (1988) argues that desire has had a pivotal place in Western thought and distinguishes two ways in which it has been understood. The first of these she associates with Plato and his understanding of desire in negative terms, as something responsive to a lack. She argues that this view of desire is dominant and continues through the work of Hegel, Freud, and Lacan. Despite differences between their positions, these thinkers all accept that desire is premised on the need to have something that is not there. The second understanding of desire she links to Spinoza and contemporary philosophers including Nietzsche, Foucault,

Deleuze, and Guattari. Within this school of thought, desire is understood as a productive force.

> In the Spinozist conception, desire is not forbidden by reality (material or cultural); on the contrary desire produces the real. It is the forces of positive production — the energy that produces things, that constructs alignments with and intersections between things, that makes. Where Hegelian Freudian desire internalises and obliterates its objects, Spinozist, or Nietzschean desire, are energies that assemble and join, separate rather than incorporate.
> (Grosz 1988:29)

In this sense, can we desire the imaginable and in so doing make it real? I am particularly interested in these issues because of my belief that part of teaching is helping students imagine their futures and constructing these as possible. And as part of this, as teachers, we need to imagine and make real a system of schooling that allows students to turn their imaginary selves into real selves. So that instead of constructing our students as lacking and our work as filling a void, we see our work as constructing alignments and intersections between students' presents and futures. In other words, we adopt the stance that Morpheas takes toward Neo.

> The act of imagination, as we have just seen, is a magical act. It is an incantation destined to make the object of one's thought, the thing one desires, appear in such a way that one can take possession of it. There is always, in that act, something of the imperious and the infantile, a refusal to take account of distance and difficulties.
> (Sartre 2004:125)

The place of the imaginary is powerful within contemporary social theory, particularly with reference to new conceptions of subjectivity associated with postmodern thought. Lacan's development of the mirror phase is pivotal to such developments. Drawing on and extending Freud's work, Lacan explains the process of identification that begins in infancy and continues through to adulthood. Through this theory, he brings into play key elements of postmodern thought including the fractured nature of subjectivity, the importance of language and the symbolic, and the significance of being located within the gaze of the Other (Grosz 1990; Sarup 1992; Fuery and Mansfield 1997).

> The *mirror stage* is a drama whose internal thrust is precipitated from insufficiency to anticipation — and which manufactures for the subject, caught up in the lure of spatial identification, the succession of fantasies that extends from a fragmented body-image to a form of its totality that I shall call orthopaedic — and, lastly, to the assumption of the armour of an alienating identity, which will mark with its rigid structure the subject's entire mental development.
> (Lacan 1997:4, original emphasis)

It is through exploration of its image in the mirror, that the infant comes to recognise, simultaneously and paradoxically, its own strengths and limitations. There is an imaginary sense of autonomy as well as a rivalry between the self, the image within the mirror and eventually the self that is projected through the gaze of others, initially the mother (perhaps also the teacher).

> The infant's mastery is in the mirror image, outside himself, while he is not really master of his movements. He only sees his form as more or less total and unified in an external image in a virtual, alienated, ideal unity that cannot actually by touched. Alienation is this lack of being by which his realisation lies in another actual or imaginary space.
> (Benvenuto and Kennedy 1986:55)

Lacan's emphasis on the imaginary and the symbolic has brought into question accepted understandings of the real. The real is not the every day but instead the space between the symbolic and the imaginary. It is linked to the desires of the unconscious as determinate of actions and reactions. In this way, 'The Real is what resists symbolisation absolutely' (Sarup 1992:112).

Because of Lacan's emphasis on the symbolic and the significance of the gaze, his theories have been applied within cultural studies to film. Not surprisingly, Zizek (2001) comments that perhaps the makers of *The Matrix* were avid readers of Lacan. Zizek discusses *The Matrix* in relation to the Lacanian notion of the Real. For him, The Matrix or 'the big Other', like every symbolic concealment, does not replace 'a real'. In this way, virtual reality is not the mechanism that turns gruel into steak and wine. Instead, the subterfuge is an attempt to conceal the void that makes reality incomplete and inconsistent. For Zizek, The Matrix is the mechanism whereby our perception of the real is distorted. In this way, The Matrix functions

> as the "screen" that separates us from the real ... However, it is here that we should not forget the radical ambiguity of the Lacanian real: it is not the ultimate referent to be covered/gentrified/domesticated by the screen of fantasy; the real is also and primarily the screen itself as the obstacle that always already distorts our perception of the referent, of the reality "out there".
> (Zizek 2001:220–221)

I am interested in exploring this notion of a screen that distorts but is nonetheless real, with regard to schooling. This will be done with reference to how students come to understand themselves and how schools come to represent themselves. These issues are interrelated. How does a 'good' school come to create 'good students' and how do 'good' students come to create a 'good school'? How is the screen that distorts our perception and camouflages the void that makes reality incomplete and inconsistent constituted when it comes to schooling? Going back to Leafy Suburbs College, I would like to argue that the scores that students gain and that facilitate their entry into elite universities are an element of this screen and that part of what this screen conceals is the students' everyday experiences of schooling. Their achievements distort our perception of their experience of schooling. In other words, as caring parents who strive to get our children into elite schools or as caring teachers who work tirelessly toward their achievement of high grades, we may not understand and acknowledge how students experience their schooling. Results may distort our perception of the referent; the reality that schooling should be a meaningful and enjoyable space for all students, a space that allows them to imagine their own futures. By teaching success, we may be enhancing, keeping in suspension, or foreclosing the act of imagination that Sartre considers as 'something of the imperious and the infantile, a refusal to take account of distance and difficulties' (2004:125).

I am also interested in the relationship between the imagined and the real as this impacts on how students see themselves and each other. Within Leafy Suburbs College, there existed common understandings about student subcultures. Groups were given names and each name was linked to behaviour, dress sense, and academic achievement. While students and staff discussed these subgroups confidently, few of the students interviewed were willing to own a label for themselves. Some would comment that they might be seen as belonging to a particular group, but this was different to seeing themselves in this way. In this sense the subculture, its label, and the behaviour assumed of it both confirmed and distorted the 'real'.

In the following chapters, I begin to provide insights into the everyday experiences of students at Leafy Suburbs College as a means of exploring this question. Before doing so, however, I will provide an overview of the academic scores achieved by students at this school and the place of Leafy Suburbs College relative to other schools. One particular interest is how this school compares to neighbourhood schools, most of which are independent and Catholic schools; and how it compares to comparable schools within the government sector. This should create a sense of 'the big Other', the mechanism through which the symbolic order related to 'good schooling' is created.

Chapter 4

Coveting a Culture of Success

On entering the website for Leafy Suburbs College, one of the first statements that opens announces that the school has a reputation for academic excellence and that there are consistently more applications for entry than places available. We are told that most students at the school aspire to university and that this aspiration is met. These statements are accompanied by an excerpt from the real estate section of a popular Melbourne newspaper. This describes how the suburb in which the school is situated includes some of the best schools in Victoria. Specific mention is made of Leafy Suburbs College, its good results, and the fact that the school zone stretches into the suburb featured. Thus we are presented with the key elements reiterated in representations of the school: academic results linked to university entry, demand outstripping supply, and entry as privilege.

A strong sense of community is evident amongst teachers, students, and parents. Taking school seriously and wanting to do well is a common priority. There is an understanding that this community of like-mindedness creates the atmosphere that in turn produces the results that make the school so in demand. 'Success stories' are talked about in the school newspapers, the school website, the neighbourhood newspapers and indeed the website announces that one of the priorities of the school is to showcase success through events such as Speech

Night. Students from the school are involved in a wide range of music, sport, and leadership programs and through these win awards including statewide awards, where they compete against the full range of schools. The school philosophy is described as offering

> a responsible and sensitive approach to education, which encourages students to achieve in a learning environment of self-discipline, mutual trust and respect. The College actively promotes a culture that encourages and celebrates the achievement of excellence. Individual diversity is valued and respected and participation by all members of the College community is encouraged. [The school] has a proud record of student achievement. The majority of students aspire to and achieve entry into university.

This culture of success is part of the history of the school and continuation of tradition forms an important element of the school ethos. There is a very active organisation of alumni, a tradition of past students returning to work at the school both as teachers and administrative staff, and students whose parents were students. Additionally, there are many teachers, including in senior positions, whose children attend the school. This inspires great confidence in the quality of the school and reiterates its reputation. The following extract is from an interview with a key member of the alumni association and illustrates a range of pertinent aspects of the school culture.

> Ten years ago in 1993, the school held a big back to the future. Because my mother is still connected to the school — the grapevine worked and I came along with a girlfriend and absolutely loved meeting up with people. The Vice Principal decided after his own school reunion that it would be good to start a similar thing in public schools because similar events generally occur in private schools. On the day of that celebration a past student started a committee and I've been involved since then. We run a reunion every year.

This alumni association also sponsors the annual awards for student excellence referred to in Chapter 1.

The education of Australian school children is divided between government and nongovernment schools, with the latter comprising systemic Catholic schools, and what are known as independent schools. Within each of these sectors there is great variation. Within the nongovernment sector there are elite Catholic and independent schools as well as parochial Catholic schools, often under-resourced. The independent sector also contains schools associated with less mainstream ethno-religious communities. In Melbourne, for example, there are Islamic, Jewish, and Greek Orthodox schools which are full-time day schools. The nongovernment sector also includes schools associated with particular pedagogies including, for example, Steiner schools. The government-sector schools charge no tuition fees per se: however, many expect payment through subject levies or what are referred to as 'voluntary contributions'. There is periodic outcry about these levies, particularly when it is revealed that schools 'punish' families who do not comply in various ways including by withholding students' reports or excluding students from some school activities until payment is received (Beauchamp 2005; Ketchell 2001; Rindfleisch 2002). Recently, there has been interest in the overall cost of government schooling in Victoria. A report indicates that parents are seeking assistance through charitable organisations in order to meet the cost of their children's schooling.

> While the "core" education remains free, the issue is over just what the "core" actually represents. Add to the extras list books, uniforms, camps, excursions and in some cases, art and music materials and computer fees — often in the guise of "voluntary levies" — and it becomes very clear that the meaning of free is a limited one.
>
> (Green 2005)

Within the nongovernment system, a wide range of fees is charged. Most Catholic schools charge modest fees, but many within the independent category charge fees considered by many to be prohibitive. Within the government sector there is also great variation. Costs associated with uniforms, books, and subject levies can make some schools quite expensive relative to others where no uniform or a modest uniform may be required and class sets of books are provided, for example. In 2004, 40% of full-time secondary students in Victoria attended nongovernment schools, including 22% who were at Catholic schools (ABS 2004). School choice is a vexed issue and for most parents it is a matter of the best available to them in the local area. Most Catholic schools remain affordable and are popular with many non-Catholic and some non-Christian parents. The preference for such schools can be responsive to perceptions of nearby government schools not being good enough, as much as perceptions about the benefits of Catholic schooling related to factors such as discipline and values.

In the context of the market, school reputation is of intense significance and in turn linked to scores achieved by students in their final year of schooling. Students in Year 12 of the Victorian Certificate of Education (VCE) strive to achieve the highest scores possible in the subjects they study to increase the number of university options open to them. Students' scores are converted into an Equivalent National Tertiary Entry Rank (ENTER), which indicates where each student is ranked in comparison to all other students. A student with an ENTER of 90.00, for example, finished ahead of about 90% of all Year 12 students. The ENTER, as an overall measure of how well a student has performed in the VCE, is the principal method of determining a student's access to university courses.

Although the Australian university sector is in a sense homogeneous, inter-institutional variations are many. There is a distinct overall pecking order of universities in attracting students to their courses. This is based on a range of factors including institutional mission, geographic location, the relative scarcity of places in courses of study offered, and student perceptions of the relative quality or reputation of the university. For universities, a key point of differentiation relates to the proportion of Year 12 high achievers attracted to each university. In Victoria, for example, the University of Melbourne attracts the highest proportion of high-achieving Year 12 students, followed by Monash University.

The significance of ENTER on university admission has led to sustained interest in how this ranking system relates to debates about social justice and education (Teese 2000). In many ways, ENTERs describe differences between groups of students or schools rather than explain why such differences occur. This is particularly pertinent with regard to debates about the relative merits of government, Catholic, and independent schools. Socioeconomic and cultural differences between students, school admission policies, and relative resourcing of schools are some of the issues that impact dramatically on relative rankings but that remain implicit in the figures.

With regard to ENTERs, school sector is a significant indicator of success. The independent school sector is far from homogeneous, comprising as it does, both high-fee, well-resourced elite schools, and schools associated with particular ethno-religious communities which may be small and relatively under-resourced, often located in poorer suburbs. Similarly the Catholic system includes some elite and relatively well-resourced schools along side others that are relatively poor, again, often linked to geographic location. Increasingly, there is also marked variation within the government sector. A strong correlation between high ENTERs, socioeconomic status, and school sector is demonstrable. The availability of the financial resources necessary to support a child through secondary education at an independent school is a key factor in explaining this correlation (Birrell et al. 2002).

The superior performance relativities of female over male students, of students from high as opposed to middle or low socioeconomic status backgrounds, and students attending independent schools rather than government or Catholic schools has been documented (Birrell et al. 2002). Some commentators argue that higher ENTERs can be produced by studying some combinations of Year 12 subjects rather than others; however, this remains controversial (Calderon, Dobson, and Wentworth 2000). Despite the proven track record of many independent schools in generating students with the highest ENTERs in the state, there has been no discussion about positive discrimination for students from relatively disadvantaged schools. This is in contrast with the UK where some commentators (Naylor and Smith 2002) are arguing that students attending particular types of schools should be given extra points.

In Australia there is no tradition of indicator data for schools being made public. It wasn't until the late 1990s that a conservative national government tested students' literacy and numeracy against a national benchmark. Victoria was the first state to make data on the VCE publicly available a few years later (Kosky 2002). The debates surrounding markets, league tables, school accountability, and effectiveness are well rehearsed in Australia as elsewhere (McGaw, Banks, and Piper 1991; Lingard, Knight, and Porter 1993; Rowe 2000; Whitty, Power, and Halpin 1998, Caldwell and Roskam 2002). At the core are concerns about the fate of public education, particularly through debates about government funding to private schools. These debates are significant and resurface regularly, particularly near elections. They reflect the historical development of Australian schooling, more or less support by particular governments for public or private schools and the place of the Catholic sector in such debates (Burke and Spaull 2001; Burke 2001). There is also ongoing debate about the possibility of such data capturing the value added of schooling relative to the social background of students. League tables are caught up in debates about markets, school effectiveness, and accountability, and in Australia there has been scepticism and resistance to something many people believe works against the grain of a tradition premised on free, secular schooling for all. Nonetheless, there are those who welcome these shifts. One commentator advocating league tables comments, 'Australian parents have more information and more rights when they buy a packet of soap powder than when they choose a school for their child' (Gannicott 1998:17–22). Those opposed to such tables argue that they work against social justice by increasing segregation. The capacity for test scores to tell us something 'real' is also contested. Economists argue that 'gaming the system', that is, enacting measures that allow some schools to do better than others by teaching to exams and, most notably, by creating opportunities to attract those students most likely to succeed, limit the utility of such tables. The main problem with using unadjusted test scores as signals of school performance is that it increases the scope for schools to game the system. Using unadjusted league tables as the principal performance indicator in a quasi-market model opens up a route for schools to improve their (perceived) performance by optimising the structure of their student body, either in terms of socioeconomic composition or prior academic ability. Furthermore, as this performance indicator is adopted by parents as a determinant of school choice, it exerts a pressure for increased social segregation between schools as student composition becomes more polarised, social segregation would obviously reduce the equity of outcomes between schools (Bradley, Draca, and Green 2004).

The Fables of Tables

In 2003, the Leafy Suburbs College newsletter announced that

> Our aim to maximise student opportunity through academic excellence has again been realised. This is attributed to the dedication of the students, the professionalism of the staff and the support of our families.

Overall scores for exit students were provided relative to the state average, student destinations were described, and top achievers showcased. It is not surprising that in the context of the market, schools aim to represent themselves in the most positive light.

It is important to note that these data do not include the results for international students. While international students are not permanent Australian residents, many undertake study in secondary schools in order to continue their studies in Australian universities. In this sense their results can be seen as relevant to the exploration being undertaken here. Further to this, there is a common-sense understanding that international, full-fee-paying students can be good for schools, not only due to the injection of funds they provide, but also because such students are understood to be 'good students' — studying diligently and achieving good results, which in turn bolster school results. Most often, international students are 'Asian' and 'Asian' is associated with being a good student. This perception of Asianness is also relevant to noninternational students and will be discussed in subsequent chapters. The initial decision to exclude international students from the data was premised on a sense of social justice as a national rather than international project. On reflection, this was a problematic starting point given globalisation and the sense of the utopian that Delors (UNESCO 1998) brings to light, discussed in Chapter 3, whereby social justice is considered in the context of globalisation. Nonetheless, had data for international students been accounted for in a coherent way, the figures below would tell a different story and one whereby each school's identity was likely to be self-evident.

The following figures situate Leafy Suburbs College relative to other comparable schools in Melbourne and to neighbourhood schools. It is based on aggregated data for university entry for 2003.

Within Melbourne, a handful of government schools achieve results comparable to those achieved at elite independent and Catholic schools. Two are single-sex and select-entry schools, taking students at Year 9 on the basis of examination. These are marked as Boys and Girls in Figure 1. Students from all sectors compete for entry to these schools and this is a process of skimming that extracts high performers from a broad range of schools, including Leafy Suburbs College. Relative to comparable government schools, Leafy Suburbs College sits mid-range, if the select entry schools are excluded.

Figures 2, 3, and 4 illustrate Leafy Suburbs College relative to schools from the government, independent, and Catholic sectors in its neighbourhood, broadly defined. The schools included are those nearby and also those understood within the school community as viable alternatives. These include some schools that are quite outside the school's surrounding area. It is not uncommon for students to travel long distances in order to attend the school of choice. In this neighbourhood, there are students who live within the zone for Leafy Suburbs College who travel long distances in order to attend an independent or Catholic school of choice, and similarly, there are students who travel very long distances in order to attend Leafy Suburbs College.

Figure 1 Leafy Suburbs College cf Elite Government Schools
– % ENTERs 80+

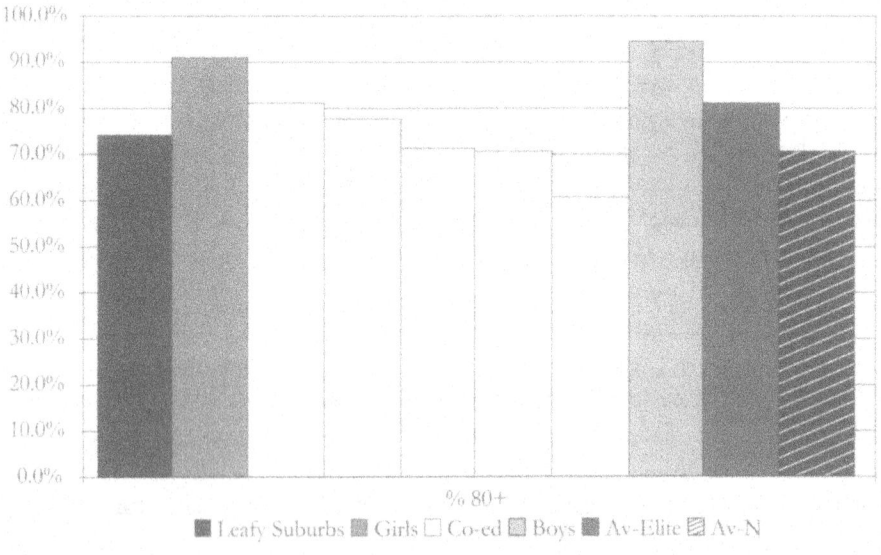

It is evident from Figure 2 that Leafy Suburbs College compares favourably to other government schools in the neighbourhood. Its students receive the highest scores and outperform the neighbourhood average.

Independent schools in the neighbourhood include elite single-sex and co-educational schools, where students receive some of the highest scores in the state. Included also are three ethno-religious schools. Jewish schools regularly produce some of the best state results and this is the case for the two from this neighbourhood. The third is a school that caters predominantly to the Greek community. This school produces the lowest results for independent neighbourhood schools. Excepting this school, independent schools produce better results than Leafy

Suburbs College. The scores between each of these schools and Leafy Suburbs College vary between 1.5% for the smallest variation to 17.7% for the highest.

There are several Catholic schools in the neighbourhood. In this category are some that would be considered local as well as two that would be considered relatively elite within this sector. One Catholic girls school does better than Leafy Suburbs College and then only by .1%.

Figure 2   Leafy Suburbs College cf Neighbourhood Other Government Schools – % ENTERs 80+

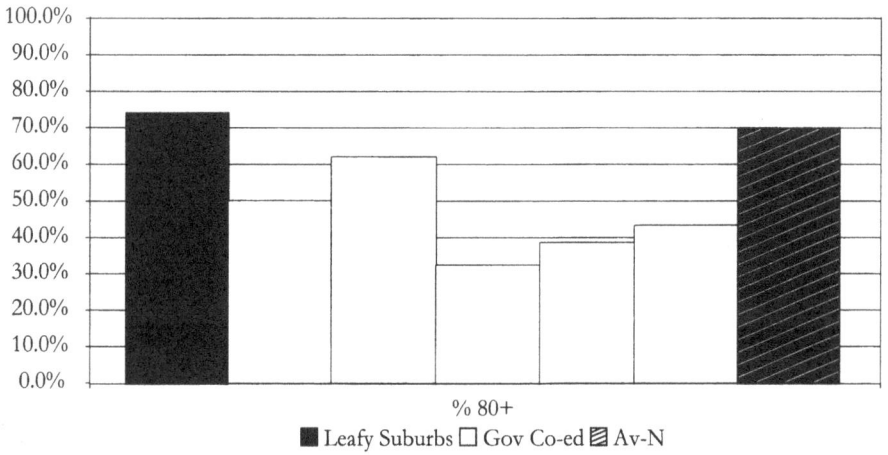

From these figures, a clearer sense can be developed of the range of issues that inform school selection. Amongst the independent schools are those that cater for specific ethno-religious communities. There are also many single-sex schools, particularly for girls, within this sector. Amongst Catholic schools there is difference related to particular religious orders and the philosophy brought through these to schooling. Single-sex schooling is more dominant within this sector, including for boys. Parents and their children may juggle a range of priorities when selecting a school and these priorities are sensitive to the perceived needs of different children within the same family. Single-sex schooling is more popular for girls than it is for boys, for example. Because of this, a family may choose a single-sex Catholic school for their daughter and a coeducational non-Catholic school for their son. Family tradition, religiosity, perceived school philosophy, family income, and identification with ethno-religious communities can be relevant factors. An active preference for government schooling also exists within some families. The ideal of a neighbourhood school that attracts a cross section of the Australian community has currency with many, but because it is perceived as the most available option, it is often constructed as a default rather than thought-through choice. Schools are increasingly configured in relation to the market and this can be a reiterative process whereby schools respond to, as well as create, particular preferences. A stark example of this is the decision by some prestigious independent boys schools to break with tradition and admit girls.

Figure 3   Leafy Suburbs College cf Neighbourhood Independent Schools – % ENTERs 80+

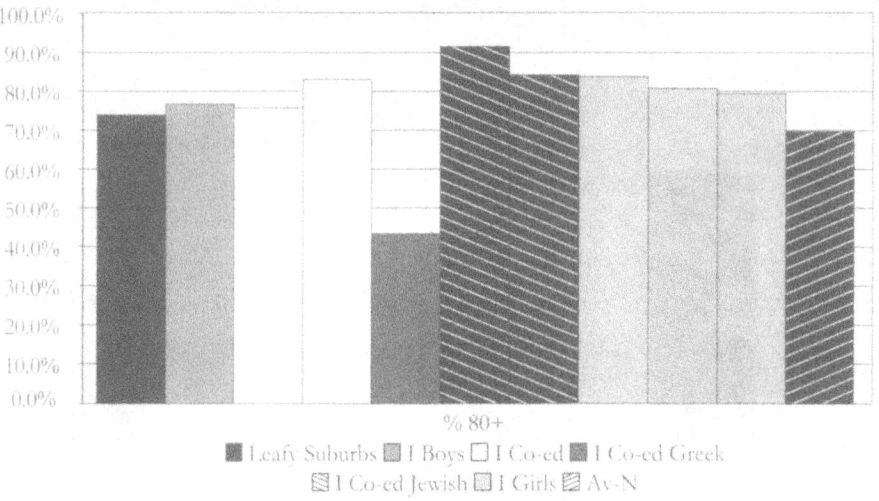

Figure 3 includes a wide range of independent schools. Some of these are ethno-religious schools including two Jewish schools and one school that caters primarily to members of the Greek community. In Melbourne there are several Jewish schools and several schools established by the Greek community that are full-time day schools. In relation to these schools, there are variations based on levels of religious orthodoxy, educational philosophy, and attitudes to language and cultural maintenance. Fee structures can also vary markedly between such schools.

In overall terms, the figures illustrate that Leafy Suburbs College compares favourably to other government schools in the neighbourhood. It is also clear that if results are the primary criteria for school choice, the high fees demanded by some of these independent and Catholic schools may not be worth paying.

Zoning In — The Politics of Entry

Academic results that facilitate university entry, high levels of demand, and entry as privilege are pivotal to the way in which Leafy Suburbs College represents itself. As indicated in the above figures, if VCE results are the major criteria for school selection, this school performs well and does so without the prohibitive fees charged by some of the nongovernment schools. Relative to neighbourhood government schools, it does extremely well even though it is not a select-entry school. These factors make obvious why there is such a high demand for places at the school. government schools like Leafy Suburbs College are most often in locations dominated by elite independent and Catholic schools. This can lead to dramatic social segregation amongst the government schools. There is also variation between the Catholic schools in the neighbourhood and this unevenness is echoed by dramatic differences in relative fee structures. Tuition fees can vary between $3,500 and $14,500 per annum between schools in the Catholic system. In the case of schools such as Leafy Suburbs College, the capacity to pay comparable fees is not a requirement for enrolment, neither is it a select-entry school. In the case of such elite government schools, the basis of enrolment can appear quite nebulous.

Figure 4   Leafy Suburbs College cf Neighbourhood Catholic Schools
– % ENTERs 80+

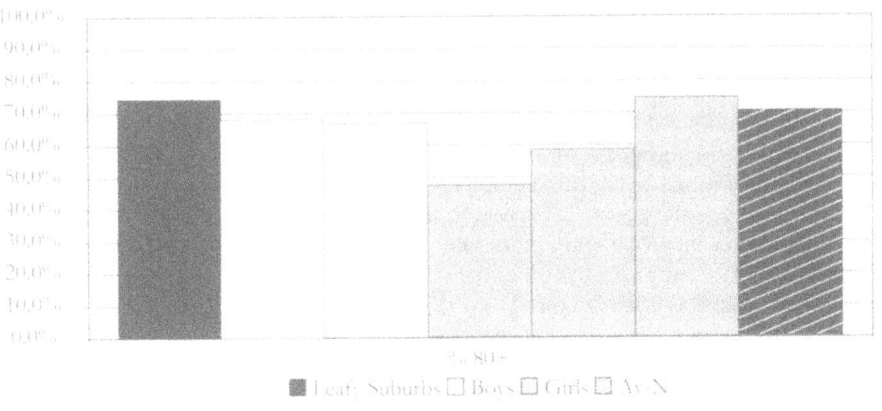

Commonly, students enter Leafy Suburbs College in three ways. Elite government schools such as Leafy Suburbs College are commonly zoned because of high demand. This means that students living within a strict geographic area are given automatic entry. However, school zone is itself a shifting category, responding to levels of demand. Siblings of enrolled students are admitted automatically. In addition, many zoned government schools have accelerated learning programs entered through examination that account for some of the enrolments. Students who live outside the zone, who do not have siblings at the school, and who have not gained a place through accelerated programs need to make a case directly to the school. Beyond strict geographic boundaries, birth sequence and exam performance, matching students and school on the basis of perceived need, and talent are laced with ambiguities and open to accusations of victimisation or favouritism. These cases are carefully argued and often supported with emotive pleas. Parents provide evidence of students' talents, including in areas such as the arts, through school reports, recommendations from primary school teachers, and evidence of additional tuition. In short, parents argue why their child will benefit from the school and in so doing, why the school will benefit from their child's attendance. The following excerpts are from interviews with mothers whose children did and did not gain a place at the school. These illustrate the depth of feeling, and in some cases, the hard work involved in getting a child into the school. At the time of the interview, the first mother quoted had a daughter in Year 10 and a daughter at primary school. Because of the sibling rule, parents will invest great effort into getting the eldest child a place, as this enables younger siblings to also attend. The next two excerpts are from interviews with mothers who applied unsuccessfully for places at the school.

> I was determined to get my daughter in. I went to every Open Day starting in Years 4, 5 and 6. I still go. It took me two years to get her in. Open Day is always crowded with people hanging outside the Hall. I always go early to get a seat. She always understood the expectation that we wanted her to go to Leafy Suburbs College. She had a letter from the principal of her primary school urging her acceptance at Leafy Suburbs College. We advised her to play an instrument other than flute, which is too popular and not as well weighted as other less popular instruments such as the oboe. She plays the flute, oboe and double bass. She does everything — she's in the school council, the debating team, she was junior captain. Students are interviewed at the end of Year 9 and nominate their VCE subjects. Students practice exams in Year 10. My daughter was practising them when she was at primary school. We told her time is essential. She was the recipient of an award last year. The school does its very best. I'll always talk up Leafy Suburbs College … what else is there? It is the best that we could afford. It does not have the resources of private schools … it has its faults … It's still a really good school. Leafy Suburbs College usually waits until the VCE results are released before hosting its Open Day. The VCE results for 2003 were not as good as 2002. The Deputy Principal is usually happy and chatting with everyone … she was very quiet this time … The Principal announced at the Information Night in 2004 that the zone will be made smaller in 2005. The Principal says that the measurement of the zone starts from the front gate.
>
> (Mother with two daughters at the school)

> I made inquiries on behalf of my daughter in 1999. I was told that my child was not eligible since I did not meet the zone requirements. I was told that I live on the wrong side of the road that marks the zone. Two students in the same class as my daughter, who do not live in the zone now attend Leafy Suburbs College. Three students from the same family living in my street attend Leafy Suburbs College.
>
> (Mother of an unsuccessful applicant)

> Her son is in the same team as the son of the Deputy Principal. Everyone from the team who applied got into Leafy Suburbs College.
>
> (Mother of an unsuccessful applicant)

These comments illustrate the intrigue that surrounds entry into Leafy Suburbs College. The pressures and consequences that surround gatekeeping are familiar in other contexts, including in relation to sought-after colleges in the United States (Steinberg 2002; Lucey and Reay 2002; Belfield and Levin 2002). However, in the case of schools such a Leafy Suburbs, these are public schools, which are supposed by many to have open access. They also illustrate the pressure students are under to succeed, the way such a system may become self-perpetuating, and how parents, students, and teachers have a vested interest in 'talking up' the school. Nonetheless, there is a paradox implicit in a process such as this. With increased demand for places, the school has more difficulty managing entry.

The Principal explained that one of the school's priorities was to juggle enrolments in response to exit numbers in order to keep the school from expanding. However, there was enormous pressure to take students and the level of demand remained unpredictable. It was difficult to predict the number and sex of siblings, for example. In the case of students within the school zone, there was a steady flow of students transferring to Leafy Suburbs College from private schools. The Principal explained that more students from private schools entered the school than Leafy Suburbs College students exited to attend such schools. Further to this, the Principal described keeping equal numbers of girls and boys a firm priority. This remained a challenge given the higher number of single-sex girls schools relative to single-sex boys schools. Juggling the numbers seemed an on going and frustrating part of the Principal's job.

There is no doubt that the school has a reputation, sometimes described as a 'culture of success'. As one member of staff stated:

> We take calls from people overseas and interstate about the school. I ask them how they did get to know about us and they'd say someone in Melbourne that I spoke to recommended Leafy Suburbs College as a good school to go to and these are people in England. They email us from there in advance of their moving saying they want their kids to go to the school. That happens on quite a regular basis either overseas or interstate — people hear about the school. Anyone can apply but acceptance criteria require that they live in the zone. We have to take families who apply who live in the zone. Anyone can apply outside of the zone — we've taken kids whose parents can't afford a private school. Leafy Suburbs College is considered the next best thing — they are attracted to its reputation. It's really hard to get into the school. We had that many people apply at the end of last year — they'd moved into the zone in January — we had to take them. It is difficult because some of the local schools have closed down. The landscape significantly impacts on the culture of the school.

Similarly, a local real estate agent described enquiries about property in the school zone received from families currently overseas and interstate. So well versed are real estate agents that one was able to recite the school zone immediately on request over the phone. The same could not be done by a Department of Education bureaucrat who instead met the request with well-choreographed avoidance. The zoning of schools such as Leafy Suburbs College is a vexed issue. Unlike select-entry schools where examination results provide transparent measures for entry, or private schools where high fees serve the same purpose, zones are nebulous, shifting and shrinking in response to increased demand. Newspapers have commented on the trend for real estate values to rise in the zones of elite government schools. Compared to similar properties outside the school zone, those within it can be up to 15% more expensive. Parents begin competing for properties when their children are toddlers for fear of being priced out of the market. There is an increasing number of families giving false addresses, bribing real estate agents to draw up false leases, and families buying properties which are sold or sublet after their children have secured a place. This has resulted in such schools conducting street checks to reveal false addresses (Tomazin 2004; Kift 2004).

Finally, however, it is the relationship between the zone and academic achievement that really matters. Is it a matter of the type of student who attends, the school culture that is effective or is it a combination of the two? A member of staff explained that the number of zoned students had increased dramatically over a number of years with between 70–80% now coming from the zone compared to 20% in previous years.

Teacher: ... when I chose the enrolments years ago, I mean I literally chose hundreds ... 225 in each year-level, I would have chosen 180 of them according to their application. So in many ways we had a huge pick of the crop, but now of course we have to take the children who are in the zone.

GT: And has that made a difference in the school?

Teacher: Not that I've noticed.

GT: So why do you think that hasn't made a difference ...?

Teacher: I think ENTER results have been going up over the last three years. Maybe teachers have got less particularly bright kids and a lot more average ones, but they make good students.

Loving and Hating the Culture of Success

Students at Leafy Suburbs College were well aware of the school's reputation for academic excellence. They understood that while this constituted a burden at one level, it was also something that would hold them in good stead into the future. In one interview, two Year 10 girls described why the school had a good reputation as follows:

Nadine: Oh, well they're going to get us money by having an education.

Amy: A good job, a good education.

Nadine: It's like a good school, it's got a pretty good reputation as well.

Amy: Teachers treat you good as well.

Nadine: We have a pretty strict uniform and they're pretty strict compared to other schools, and there's not many druggies compared to other schools. So you don't really see many people with slicked back blonde hair with black regrowth and eye makeup everywhere. If you see someone like that you'd think 'Oh what school do they go to?'

GT: How do you think the school compares with others?

Nadine: I think it's pretty good … actually our school's not very nice to look at! But yeah, compared to the schools in the area the facilities aren't as good as some of them, but overall, the results we get are probably a lot better than the other public schools in the area.

GT: Why do you think that?

Nadine: Um, I dunno.

Amy: They push hard on us to do well.

Nadine: Yeah, the people here that actually want to learn, they actually want to get an education and that sort of influences other people around them for them to want to do good. Whereas, at some other schools people just don't care, and because they don't, that influences on everyone.

Another girl who had transferred to Leafy Suburbs College from a Catholic girls' school felt that at her previous school 'you can get away with a lot of things, and not do work and get away with it. At Leafy Suburbs College I never could, so it's different in that way'. In a similar vein, another interviewee commented that at Leafy Suburbs College the teachers

> like to keep you on track with your work, like, don't want you to miss anything and they always want you to hand things in and stuff. It's annoying sometimes, because you always have to be on track, but it's good in a way, because they really want you to try — they want you to do well in that subject. Whereas sometimes other schools I hear about they're not … it doesn't get to them as much that people are falling behind because it's their own choice, whereas Leafy Suburbs College on your back forcing you to do your best — well not forcing you but encouraging you. (Lucy)

It is worth visiting the words of past students. Had the school delivered what was promised? How, as adults, did they view their education at the school?

Nick, a forty-six-year-old accountant, had attended Leafy Suburbs College. He left the school in his final year, prior to sitting the exams. He did not look back on his years at Leafy Suburbs College with particular fondness. He commented that

> There was no attempt at the end of Term 1 1976 when I was in Form 6 [Year 12] to correct my poor grades. I was basically told there was no future for me. In essence the school was not interested in students that may have adversely affected their results. The school was renown for good results through actively weeding out students they felt may not pass and pass well. I have often thought about my experience at Leafy Suburbs College and now believe that had the school been more focused on the students rather than the results, the results may well have been as good if not better.

Close to thirty years later, interviewees make comments laced with similar sentiments. A member of staff described the same mechanism for success.

> They're counselled out before they fail, even if that's halfway through Year 12! I would change the policy that the numbers matter the most.

The Cost of Community and Its Imagined Style

> It's a great school. I have problems with its conservatism, in terms of uniform and diversity and I don't want to look at a future of Australia where it relies on scores and marks and grades. And it advocates that you need to afford to go to the school — because it's public education, it should accept everyone and try with everybody. So that's the only thing I find a problem here, but given that, it's really easy. The kids are beautiful, and I think they're beautiful because there's a sense of community and belonging here. Perhaps because it creates an exclusive community everyone feels ... once you're in Leafy Suburbs College you feel like you belong. But it's really hard to get into Leafy Suburbs College and you're kind of pushed out if you're different.

This statement, made by a member of staff captures the paradox of community. Its benefits rely on its capacity to exclude. Its identity relies on sameness. Anderson reminds us that communities are imagined and 'distinguished, not by their falsity/genuiness, but by the style in which they are imagined' (Anderson 2003:6). The imagined style of Leafy Suburbs College community relies on a like-mindedness related to academic achievement. Regardless of your background or your income, you are part of the community because you take school seriously, wish to succeed, and will do your best in order to achieve the results for which the school is famous. While some staff argue that there has been a shift over the years regarding the politics of entry, there is still pressure on enrolled students to perform in the style imagined appropriate for this community. Of course, academic aspiration and achievement are not equally distributed and again Anderson's comment with reference to the imagined community of nation has a particular salience in this context. He states:

> it is imagined as a community, because, regardless of the actual inequality and exploitation that may prevail in each, the nation is always conceived as a deep, horizontal comradeship.
>
> (Anderson 2003:7)

In a similar way, Leafy Suburbs College is imagined as bereft of actual inequality. Instead, an ethos of meritocracy prevails whereby students' achievements reflect their efforts and natural talents as though these could be determined quite independently of social background. In the remainder of this chapter this imagined community will be explored with particular reference to class and ethnic difference.

The Loud Silence of Class

A neatly dressed young man handed me a champagne flute that contained half a strawberry suspended on a bed of bubbles. Trios of musicians filled the air with subtle music while other students offered tasty finger food from large silver platters. It was the opening night of the school art show and the specialist science wing had been transformed into a gallery for the occasion. At each turn the visitors were faced with a roomful of sculpture, drawing, painting, or folios from graphic communications classes. These rooms were brimming with excited faces, the students themselves and of course their parents and teachers. Eventually we were ushered into the library for the announcement of this year's winners. Students were nominated from each year-level as worthy of commendation. One of the local real estate agents supported the show by providing a prize for the piece of art judged best by an expert and this piece would be hung in the school foyer. The large billboard outside the school gates announcing the event was emblazoned with the name and logo of the real estate office.

In Victoria there is great variation between schools within the Catholic, independent, and government sectors. There is also great variation within each of these sectors. The private/public divide whereby private schools are positioned as wealthy and public schools as poor, resonates but tells a limited story. Commonly, such characterisations are built on comparisons between the elite independent and Catholic schools and some of the poorer government schools. This is a contentious issue and is regularly and vehemently debated, particularly with reference to government funding formulas. The comparisons can be stark even in the same suburb, with students from relatively humble schools aware of neighbourhood schools that are well endowed with grand buildings, playing fields, and facilities such as theatres, chapels, and halls. In this context, the basis for comparison becomes important. At Leafy Suburbs College, students and staff are aware that relative to many other government schools, theirs is a well-resourced school, but in comparison to some of the independent and Catholic schools, their school is found seriously lacking. In this sense, being an elite government school that functions within the ballpark of well-performing schools makes such comparisons starker. Most government schools are not part of this competition.

Students had a strong sense of their school's place as a 'good' government school and linked this to academic results. Some understood this as teachers pushing them to perform. Some students had a strong sense of the entanglement of issues around funding, resources, and academic achievements. In some cases, students linked these complex interrelationships to what they did not like about their school. In one exchange between two students, the school was described as 'mercenary' and this was explained with reference to these issues.

Daniel: The way they look at students I think, and the way they look at getting your money in as if money is more important than anything really! I don't know what it's like in other schools, because every school needs money and I realise that, but I do think this school takes a particularly hard line on getting your money in, and getting the fees in.

Stephen: Well, they do, because one of the selection criteria for getting into Year 7 is past academic achievements and the ability to play a musical instrument, so obviously if you're a good academic you might win awards and stuff for the school, which generates money for them.

Daniel: It generates prestige, more than money.

Stephen: That too, which gives them, well, they can get grants from the government and stuff for being a good school.

Daniel: We do get grants.

Stephen: Exactly, so that's one thing that they have.

Leafy Suburbs College is situated in one of Melbourne's 'leafy' suburbs. 'Leafy' is a euphemism for comfortable, often denoting being middle-class rather than affluent. Nonetheless, such suburbs can be sandwiched between significantly wealthy and distinctly less wealthy neighbouring suburbs. Because of this, a school like Leafy Suburbs College can enrol students from a wide range of socioeconomic backgrounds and it became evident during the course of this study that there were families at the school who were struggling to meet the financial burden of their children's schooling. As has been discussed, the cost of attending a government school can vary enormously because of marked variations in subject levies, so-called voluntary contributions, uniform, and book costs. Leafy Suburbs College would be considerably more expensive than many government schools. Interviewees claimed that families were 'hounded' if they did not pay school levies, even though a case for exemption could be made. In one infamous case, a family was asked to justify their claim that the levies were beyond them, after their child paid to attend a school camp the previous year. If they could afford the camp, it was argued, they could afford the levies. The family withdrew their child from the school the following year.

During interviews, the issue of poverty, with specific reference to 'Australian' students was raised. Such students were referred to as the children of 'battlers' who were sometimes seen as struggling in a school considered to assume middle-class values and attributes. One teacher described 'Australian' as 'fifth-generation Australian kids with no money'. This was further elaborated:

> … the kids who are socioeconomically disadvantaged. They're the kids who are really Australian, not the ones who are from other countries … they're a really small group and they often feel excluded. They're the kids who can't afford new shoes and yet they're hounded about not having school shoes.

Another teacher commented that there were 'quite a few' families at the school who received the Government Education Maintenance Allowance (EMA) commonly understood as an indicator of poverty.

> [In one year-level] we've got at least ten kids who haven't paid subject contribution fees out of about fifty, partly because they're on EMA.

It was argued that socioeconomic status was the 'biggest hurdle' at the school where middle-class values dominated. Most parents were professionals, most students aspired to higher education, and most families had the income that was commonly associated with these aspirations. This created

> a sense of exclusivity and a bit of snobbery and arrogance goes along with the middle-class attitude we have here, as in 'I go to Leafy Suburbs College and therefore I don't go to a working-class suburb school'. I think there's that. The dominant culture of the school is middle-class, higher achiever, which is good, but I try and bring in material from different places to get the kids to understand that not everyone lives with the privileges they live with.

Mining the Migrant Mentality

In Australia, determining class can be problematic, particularly with reference to educational aspirations and parental agency. How the working-class is constituted and how educational achievement is tracked in relation to it become increasingly slippery, particularly when ethnic background is put into the mix. Within discussions of class, cultural diversity can be ignored or constituted separately by naming it as a distinct category. The above comments about the 'Aussie battler' illustrate a common-sense view that constitutes the working-class as white, 'real' Australian and most often male. The corollary is the constitution of 'ethnic' communities as middle-class by default. Such communities either were middle-class prior to migration or have high aspirations that will translate into upward social mobility. These narratives about migrants shift in relation to particular communities and the time of migration, but there are some common features. Education is linked to ambition, a desire for children to experience better lives than those of their parents. There is a narrative that links it to parents who want their children to achieve what they were denied. This is about education linked to status as much as to economic acceleration. There is also a view that links the valuing of education, in its own right, with particular cultures. Such narratives often intermingle and also cross-pollinate with other more general views about migrants. They can do more with less because they are accustomed to deprivation. An alternative work ethic that extends to scholastic effort is associated with some migrant groups. This is used to explain why people from such communities will sacrifice lifestyle in order to get ahead. For the Chinese in particular, this alternative work ethic is understood as one of the elements that contributes to their success. These are the students who others describe as not having a life because they spend their time studying. Alternatively, there are groups, such as the Turks and the Lebanese, who are characterised as not valuing education, particularly for women. For some groups, education can be seen as an embedded cultural element such as in the case of Russian Jews or the Chinese (Tsolidis 2001; Archer and Francis 2005; Rapoport and Lomsky-Feder 2002).

At the most basic level, however, data used to track educational achievement can be insensitive to ethnicity. While place of birth is a transparent category in the data, it may not tell us about language spoken, itself tenuously linked to ethnic identification. And in the long term, there is increased fuzziness around such categories due to language loss, mixed marriages, and multiple migrations, which lessen the possibility of meaningful collection and interpretation of the data used to explore educational inequality. As Teese and Polesel comment with regard to their own work,

> While the area-based methodology of assigning socioeconomic status to individuals does bring out the relationship between aspirations and social position, it is insensitive to key individual differences, in this case a family history of migration and the high place accorded to academic learning amongst certain immigrant groups, such as the Chinese and Vietnamese.
>
> (Teese and Polesel 2003:168)

Over a quarter of students attending Leafy Suburbs College were born overseas and in most cases, these students spoke a language other than English at home, most commonly one of the Chinese languages or Russian. This reflects patterns of immigration as much as anything else. However, both these groups are associated with high educational achievement. It is highly likely that these groups of students would benefit the school because they and their families take education very seriously. The students who were the children or grandchildren of immigrants, however, were not associated with educational achievement so unambiguously. In the case of those with Greek or Italian backgrounds, they were struggling to maintain a foothold at the school.

In the case of students attending elite government schools, family aspirations and their link to migration may be a significant issue. Prohibitive fees charged by elite independent and Catholic schools may encourage relatively newly arrived families for whom such schooling is a priority, to seek enrolment at elite government schools. Similarly, students may travel from an uncharacteristically wide range of addresses to attend such schools. Additionally the neighbourhoods such schools are part of are themselves diverse. At an anecdotal level, there are stories of immigrant families renting small flats near such schools in order to gain enrolment, while the large and relatively luxurious family homes in the vicinity house students who attend elite independent and Catholic schools. Schools like Leafy Suburbs College are attractive to immigrant families with high aspirations for their children and in turn, such schools find these students attractive. Staff and students at Leafy Suburbs College understand immigrant students with Chinese and East European backgrounds to be high achievers. Because of this, their priorities are judged as a means of maintaining the school's reputation for academic excellence. Despite their relative recency of arrival, they are not always associated with economic deprivation. One member of staff explained with reference to the Russian community,

> Leafy Suburbs College, of course, has a huge Russian population. They're mostly Jewish. And so they've got a double sense of community as soon as they arrive in Australia, not only are they accepted but also I'm sure they're helped quite substantially financially, by that community. They don't seem hard-done by.

How particular ethnic groups are constructed vis-à-vis educational attainment is a controversial issue. These often rely on stereotypes of what it means to be 'Russian', 'Jewish', 'immigrant' or 'Chinese'. Further to this, such debates are caught up with arguments about the impact of immigrant aspirations and how these may be maintained by the so-called second generation. I have argued elsewhere (Tsolidis 2001) that the likelihood of particular immigrant communities maintaining the value added by the aspirations associated with migration varies.

While there were indications that the children of Greek immigrants, for example, were well represented in university figures relative to their socioeconomic peers, this has not been maintained. However, the same may not be the case for other groups, including the Russians and Chinese. These issues are caught up in debates about national belonging as much as anything else. There is a xenophobic view that 'Australian' cannot naturally or effortlessly extend beyond those with a British heritage. In this context, there is relatively little focus on British immigration and on the other hand, a long history of focusing on the Chinese as alien to and threatening of the Australian lifestyle (Castles et al. 1988; Vasta and Castles 1996, Hage 1998, 2003). In this context, understanding who gains access to highly sought-after university places is filtered through Australia's national imaginary, which can nuance particular groups' success or failure very differently.

Is Anything Really Priceless?

> As everyone knows, priceless things have their price, and the extreme difficulty of converting certain practices and certain objects into money is only due to the fact that this conversion is refused in the very intention that produces them, which is nothing other than the denial (Verneinung) of the economy.
>
> (Bourdieu 1977)

In this study, entry into universities, particularly those understood as elite, is taken to indicate educational success. In Australia, the classification of universities as more or less elite is linked to the scores needed by students to be offered a place, particularly in prestigious courses such as medicine or law. This process is far from benign and reflects the reproductive nature of education, one that has been consolidated through the infatuation with markets in Australia as elsewhere (Marginson 1997). In this context, it is not surprising that class as a sociological category has re-emerged as a significant way of understanding education. Connell (2003) argues that the 'hidden injuries' of class are consistent in studies conducted in the UK, United States, and Australia and go some way to explaining the persistence of educational inequality. He argues that working-class parents exhibit scepticism about schooling, which is manifest in their relationships with schools and teachers. Connell suggests that while the explanatory power of 'cultural capital' is limited, its usefulness lies in the impetus it provides for examination of family background and relations between families, communities, and schools. The concepts of 'cultural capital' and 'cultural deprivation' 'suggest, specifically, that the attitudes and aspirations of parents might be important influences on how children relate to schooling, and ultimately, how schools function' (Connell 2003:229).

There are well over one thousand students enrolled at Leafy Suburbs College Of the students enrolled, close to 73% were born in Australia. The remaining students were born in forty-four different countries, with the largest groups coming from China, Russia, and the Ukraine. Over 80% of the school population nominated English as the language spoken at home. The languages, other than English, most commonly spoken at home were Chinese and Russian; however, twenty-eight different languages were named. Close to 70% of the school population lived within the immediate school area. However, other students came from sixty-four suburbs from a staggeringly wide range of areas. Included were some of the poorest and wealthiest areas of Melbourne and in the case of some students, they were travelling between twenty and thirty kilometres in order to reach the school from their home.

The link between place of residency, family background, academic aspirations, and achievements is not straightforward. In this sense, when a school such as Leafy Suburbs College is described as middle-class, we need to consider what is being characterised as such. It may be the students and their families, the suburb, or the school ethos, itself a nebulous thing. Which of these elements is primary, if any, in allowing students to gain university entry? In other words, there may be something in the mix that is genuinely priceless. What is the 'social magic' that allows a school that represents itself as 'good' to become such, even when the students come from diverse social backgrounds? The students from Leafy Suburbs College who make it to university may be those Bourdieu (1988) describes as the 'the lucky survivors' of a system whereby their success is not typical of their peers. Is it a case of excellent mimesis — of students from a range of backgrounds, with a range of beliefs and experiences adapting en masse to the doxa of symmetry between middle-classness and educational achievement? Butler reminds us that Bourdieu's view of mimesis 'works almost always to produce a conformity or congruence between the field and the *habitus*, the question of ambivalence at the core of practical mimeticism — and, hence, also in the very *formation* of the subject — is left unaddressed (Butler 1999:119, original emphasis). It is this ambivalence at the core of subjectivity and how it plays out through student subcultures that will be explored further in following chapters. However, this ambivalence is played out through the matrix of relations, discourses, and structures that are provided through Leafy Suburbs College.

Leafy Suburbs College was characterised by some as a 'pretend private' school. This was illustrated with reference to its strict uniform code, the expectation that parents pay fees, the high academic standards, and linked to this, the more limited curricula on offer. Students also had access to a range of music, art, science, and technology facilities that were not available at all government schools. Perhaps more than these issues, there was the argument that emphasised the politics of enrolment. The school succeeded because it was able to attract the type of students most likely to achieve the academic results on which it built its reputation. This was done through a set of entry requirements tagged to particular curriculum areas. These were variously understood as either a filtering mechanism aimed at keeping 'nonachievers' out or a system that allowed students with particular aptitudes the opportunity to succeed. These are complex issues that lie at the heart of debates about schooling and social justice. Here, the aim is to provide insights from within a government school that is cast as a 'pretend private' school. The argument explored is that when education is a market, the positioning of some government schools as elite creates both strength and vulnerability. It is a fragile privilege that in many ways creates a heavy burden for teachers, students, and parents. It speaks of the ambiguity that is present in all 'in-between spaces', that of simultaneous entrapment and empowerment.

Chapter 5

Strategic Identities — Pathways to Imagined Futures

> The school tends to focus a lot on numbers and how many people get into uni and which uni, and the scores that they get in Year 12, and unfortunately it's a bit contradictory because the whole system of course — secondary education — relies on numbers and statistics and it is really important that we get those higher marks because those kids will receive the course that they want to, if they do really well. However, I think that there's something lost in that ideological framework, in that you've got to spend more time making kids be better people, feel good about themselves, feel good about society, it's not just about grades and marks. Leafy Suburbs College is probably more interested in grades and marks and appearances and superficiality than it should be, but given that that's how to succeed in our society then unfortunately that's the way it is. (Teacher)

> Identity is a simultaneous struggle against dissolution and fragmentation; an intention to devour and at the same time a stout refusal to be eaten ...
>
> (Bauman 2004:77)

The population of Leafy Suburbs College is diverse. At the time of the study, students enrolled had been born in forty-four different countries, spoke twenty-eight different languages, and lived in seventy different suburbs. These suburbs included some of the wealthiest and poorest in Melbourne, with some students living twenty to thirty kilometres away from the school. Yet there was a sense of community at the school that was steeped in like-mindedness about the value of education. I have argued that in some ways this is an imagined community that relies on exclusion — a politics of enrolment that allows those most likely to succeed to enter and a system of counselling that encourages those unlikely to succeed to leave. The overall aim here is to consider how this imagined community is experienced by students in relation to processes of identification that are steeped in ambivalence. Leafy Suburbs College is one of very few government schools that facilitates students' entry into elite universities. Their success is a product of what makes their school elite within the government sector, but also illustrates how, in order to achieve, a school like Leafy Suburbs College has to do more with less. This places huge pressure on students, staff, and parents and, in many ways, positions them as both privileged and vulnerable. Perhaps it is a process of what Pope (2001) describes as 'doing school' — a system that encourages students to do well, rather than to experience education.

> They [students] realise that they are caught in a system where achievement depends more on 'doing' — going through the correct motions — than on learning and engaging with the curriculum. Instead of thinking deeply about the content of their courses and delving into projects and assignments, the students focus on managing the work load and honing strategies that will help them to achieve high grades.
>
> (Pope 2001:4)

Here, I wish to begin to explore the identities that students bring to the task of 'doing school'. How do they as adolescents reconcile who they are within the culture of a school where sameness is assumed and yet great difference also exists? This exploration will be framed in relation to student subcultures.

Students and staff at Leafy Suburbs College described particular subcultures that operated within the school. Common labels were used and there was also agreement about their benign nature relative to those assumed to operate at other schools. These groups were not seen as threatening the harmony that existed at Leafy Suburbs College nor were such groups understood as hard edged. Instead, they illustrated special interests rather than tribal or combative groupings. Nonetheless, membership of particular groups was understood as more or less coveted. Membership of some groups was attributed readily, linked variously to ethnic origins and embodiment. Membership of other groups came as a result of hard work. Entry into 'the popular kids' or 'cool kids' was the most difficult, sometimes requiring high intrigue. Being identified as a 'nerd' or 'geek', on the other hand, required hard work of a different kind, excelling or at least aspiring to academic excellence. The other groups identified included the 'wogs', the 'musos', the 'Goths', the 'Asians', the 'Russians', the 'hardcores', the 'blonde' girls, and the 'jocks'.

Group membership is linked to a real and imagined choice. How you look, where you were born, what type of family you belong to predetermine how difficult it is for you to enter or exit particular groups. Skeggs (2004) argues that cosmopolitanism is a middle-class marker allowing a playfulness in relation to identity not available to the working-classes within which the making of self is not possible. Instead, the working-classes just 'are'. In this context, how real are students' identity choices? One of the most intriguing aspects of working with the students at the school was the way they identified subcultures with certainty and yet, with as much certainty claimed that they did not fit into any one of the groups they identified. In this way, these subcultures belonged to others, never to those who named them. Thus there was an ambivalence of belonging.

Bauman makes the point that this ambivalence is part of liquid modernity. There is a simultaneous need for and rejection of friendship, love, and community. On the one hand, these provide much-needed security in times of uncertainty, and on the other hand, in so doing, restrict our capacity to develop the transient identities increasingly requisite. 'Identities are for wearing and showing, not for storing and keeping' (Bauman 2004:89).

Here, the overall contention is that students at Leafy Suburbs College were getting lived experience in wearing and showing identities through these school subcultures. Ultimately students' capacity to move within and between these subcultures linked to the futures they imagined and their capacities to achieve such futures. Whilst it is important to acknowledge student agency, it also needs to be understood as responsive to structures, in this context those provided by an elite Government school. Leafy Suburbs College has been categorised as 'elite' relative to other Government schools. By comparison to public schools in its neighbourhood, the results are better, the facilities are better, and it is zoned because more students want entry than places available. The school offers a tighter and narrower rendition of academic culture than other neighbourhood public schools. Arguably, what it offers is also narrower than that offered at many of its neighbourhood Independent and Catholic schools where better resources support a greater breadth of offerings. Some staff, parents, and students involved in this study described the school's academic culture as an unidimensional interpretation, whereby scores, university entry, and the subjects that best facilitate these were the only things highlighted. Such an environment is experienced as more or less oppressive by various groups of students. However, it also serves to sharpen identity choices and their consequences for students. Students have to learn to do more with less, to become more strategic with their identifications. In this section, the student subcultures will be described. The overall aim is to consider how these were characterised by students and staff at the school and how they were understood in relation to academic success. This provides an overview for the discussion to follow which will consider how particular students situated themselves in relation to these subcultures.

The 'popular' kids were the most revered by staff and students. In many cases they were all-round high achievers. Many had leadership qualities, most obvious in relation to sport or music. They mentored younger students and were social, 'life of the party' types. They were the faces you came to recognise through attendance at Speech Nights, art award nights, music concerts, theatre, and in the photographs that adorned the school foyer showcasing students' achievements outside school. While individuals within this group may have excelled in a specific field such as music, they nonetheless appeared at the school sports or in the debating teams. They were the sort of student you wanted your own daughter or son to become and they were the type of student many teachers clearly enjoyed having in their classes and being involved with during extracurricular activities. These students congealed into a group in junior-year levels and travelled through their school years as a tight-knit group. Parents recognised each other from the multitude of deliveries and pickups from houses where these students congregated on Saturday or Friday nights. Here, loud music, 'must have' outfits, relationships, and eventually alcohol and cigarettes earmarked membership. Intrigue linked to friendship and girl/boy relationships, particularly amongst the girls, earmarked membership. Students from this group set the benchmark for what was fashionable and the approach to appearance was labour intensive. In a school where strict uniform code operated, the 'must have' look was displayed on the weekend and at school in subtle ways. At school, such students sported the latest hairstyles. Nonetheless, the look cultivated was subdued elegance, which was differentiated from loud or stand-out haircuts and colour.

At the other end of the spectrum were the students most commonly described as 'nerds'. The 'nerds' or 'geeks' were those students who excelled academically but were seen to do so at the expense of having a social life. In everyday Australian parlance they were 'daggy' rather than fashionable or 'cool'. Most often these were the students in accelerated learning programs. Within this group there was variation, particularly amongst the boys. Their interests were caricatured to include science fiction, computer games, and hobbies such as War Hammer. These were not the 'sporty' boys, but instead those who played chess, table tennis, or 'four square' or down ball (a no-contact ball game). While such students may have played musical instruments, they were more likely to be strings in the orchestra than brass in the various ensembles inspired by jazz. Unlike the sporty 'jocks', macho 'wogs' and 'popular' boys, their masculinity was more amorphous and less stridently identified with heterosexual relationships.

Because of the association with academic excellence, there was a clear overlap between the 'nerds', the 'Asians' and the 'Russians' at this school. 'Asian' was used to describe students from a range of ethnicities and birthplaces, including international students who were in Australia to complete courses and living with guardians. However, many students in this category were ethnically Chinese, including those whose families had been in Australia for many years and others who may have been born in Hong Kong or Taiwan, for example. In a similar way, 'Russians' was used to capture students who were born in a range of places within Eastern Europe. However, most in this category were born overseas. In Australia, as elsewhere, the Chinese and Russians are associated with academic excellence. In part this is because of the link often made between migration and educational aspirations (Portes and Rumbaut 2001; Khoo et al. 2002; Birrell and Khoo 1995). Nonetheless, the same link is not made for all immigrant groups. What it means to be Chinese or Russian, particularly Jewish Russian, is linked to cultural traits that are stereotypically associated with education for each group. For the Chinese, this is commonly tagged to discipline, diligence, and parents who demand a great deal from their children (Archer and Francis 2005; Tsolidis 2000). The amorphous term 'Asian' was used by students with reference to a group of 'Asian looking' students regardless of their place of origin, length of Australian residency, and self-identification. Like the term 'wog', 'Asian-ness' has a strong history in Australia concerned with migration and related policy. Debates surrounding immigrants from Southeast Asia go back to the Gold Rushes and policies of exclusion such as the white Australia policy. These debates resurface with unforgiving regularity in relation to foreign policy, immigration, and so-called border protection. With reference to education and schooling, 'Asian' students are sometimes constructed as a threat because of their assumed work ethic and determination to excel. At Leafy Suburbs College, some students referred to such students and their capacity for hard work rather than talent. This characterisation was exemplified by the description of the divide between those doing classical music and those doing other forms of music. Those doing classical music were described as mainly 'Asians' who practised for hours and had excellent technique as a result. On the other hand, other forms of music emphasised interpretation in ways that afforded non-Asian students the chance to excel. The significance of this representation of Chinese-ness is how it sits vis-à-vis racist discourses, particularly those linked to education as a limited resource. In the context of such discourses, the Asian student is constructed as a threat in what Hage (1998) describes as the neurotic imaginary. Here superhuman attributes are used to dehumanise 'Asians', a form of racism that relies on positive rather than negative representations.

Many of the 'Russians' at Leafy Suburbs College were Jewish. It has been argued that the notion of 'intelligentsia' is central to the Russian Jewish ethnic identity and includes as high priorities the learning of musical instruments, studying of literature, particularly canonical Russian literature, and aspirations for university education. Strong family and community ties are critical in transferring and sustaining this sense of identity. Arguing in relation to Israel, Rapoport and Lomsky-Feder make the following comment:

> The notion of intelligentsia is embodied in being a Russian Jew and provides the immigrants with a conceptual-and-identity anchor in any social space they inhabit. As the generative, personal, and collective, capital embedded in Russian Jewish space, intelligentsia links the subjective world of the individual Russian Jew to the social and cultural world she/he inhabits.
>
> (Rapoport and Lomsky-Feder 2002:235)

Not all the Jewish students at the school were Russian and not all Russians were Jewish; however, Jewishness was associated with strong academic aspirations by some of the teachers interviewed. As one teacher put it, 'the Jewish community, as a religious group or a cultural group or whatever, do take learning more seriously'. The Russian Jews, in particular, were associated with a strong community that provided them with support. While 'Asian' students were also linked to academic achievement, comments made by staff and students did not link them with a similar sense of community.

The 'blonde' girls and the 'jocks' were terms used by research participants to describe those students who were seen as unlikely to excel academically and who were struggling to stay at the school past Year 10. They played cricket and Australian-rules football, used skateboards, and surfed. They were most often 'real' Australians who had a good time in 'down to earth' ways. These were the children of parents who accused others of putting on airs. The girls were characterised as being accessories to the boys. These were the students who spent their summers at the swimming pool; the boys were good-looking lifeguards while the girls were simply good looking. Their social life often centred on the local footy club or cricket club. Here, parents helped to create a cross-generational community through fund-raising, coaching, and support for players. Finals and annual events such as award nights involved a wider group of students from the school. There was some overlap between the 'popular' kids and these students; however, the major difference seemed to be that the 'blondes' and 'jocks' were not considered academically competent nor as investing heavily in music, art, or theatre. Instead, this group was sometimes constructed as functioning within the margins of a school that assumed middle-class values and lifestyle. Some staff were less pessimistic about this group and instead constructed them as the 'sporty-cool-dude kids' who through sport, showed leadership skills essential within the school. Over the period of the study there had been instances where students from such families had been counselled to leave the school. One mother described how she had to insist that her son had the right to remain at the school, despite achieving marks in Year 10 considered unacceptably low by the school. He was a star cricket player and footballer. His sister, however, left the school at the end of Year 10. Such families relayed stories laced with resentment and sometimes turned their backs on a school they considered constructed their families 'as not good enough' with the possible exception of prowess on the cricket field or football oval. For some of these families there was also the issue of the cost of schooling and what was described by some interviewees as the 'hounding for levies'.

The 'musos' were students who were seen as distinctly talented. These students attended to alternative cultural mores such as jazz music and European film. They revelled in being intelligently different. Rather than commercial fashion brands, they wore clothes that made bold, countercultural statements. There was a quiet belligerence about their stance. The 'musos' were heavily involved in the school music program and in playing music in bands outside the school. Some had experienced success as artists outside the school. Key 'musos' congregated at various clubs and pursued their musical interests, including with others who did not attend the school. The 'musos' were involved in school events such as concerts, but their participation had an air of benevolence about it — a realisation that a particular type of performance was 'not cool' but good for the school. In a reciprocal fashion, the school seemed more tolerant of seemingly aberrant behaviour, for example, the wearing of what in other circumstances would be classified as 'extreme' and therefore unacceptable hairstyles.

The 'musos' were also a form of elite within the school. The music program was extensive with students being withdrawn from regular classes to have specialist tuition. Additionally, there existed a wide array of performance groups that needed to be accommodated with the weekly timetable. For some teachers, this constituted an imposition.

> I'd do something about the music program. Because ... we have to arrange classes at Year 7 according to music, strings, Languages Other Than English, English as a Second Language, it makes a really tight formation of classes and that also impacts further up the years. Like I'd do something about music, because they've all got to be according to the different classes but if they had their band practice before school and it didn't impact on curriculum that would open up and give us so much freedom. That's something I would change but it's too hard to change the music faculty.

While this teacher describes many impositions on the timetable, music is the one targeted and furthermore assumed to be the most resistant to change. In some people's mind, the music program was a euphemism for a system that streamed the top achievers. Another member of staff commented:

'they're the 'music kids', but the music kids are the ones who apply themselves with academic rigor. And the others — they're at the bottom of the barrel.

In Australia, it is the 'wogs' who play soccer, whose brothers drive the elaborately painted and noisy cars, and who listen to disco and rap music. There is a history of migration and the alienation that is part of this, implicit in the term 'wog'. The term was used to ridicule newly arrived southern European immigrants in the 1960s and 1970s. In the 1980s the term was popularised by comedians through so-called ethnic humour. More recently, 'wog' has become a form of strident self-identification, used with pride by the grandchildren of immigrants. There is persistent debate about who has the right to use it and by implication allowed into a community whose identity has been forged, more or less, as a reaction to xenophobia. The term is linked to migration but not all migrants are accepted as 'wogs'. Most commonly it is associated with post–World War II migration from southern Europe; increasingly, there is debate about the place of those from Turkey and the Middle East within this category (http://www.wog.com.au/article_main.asp?ArticleId=416).

At Leafy Suburbs College, the 'wogs' were students whose grandparents had migrated from Italy and Greece in the 1960s and 1970s. In one teacher's terms, these were 'the soccer boys' who took pride in their Greek or Italian heritage and in being 'wogs'. Describing some boys in his class, he commented:

> Yeah, I'm Greek and we're doin' the Olympics. There's very much a sense of pride in that. But again it's on a very small scale compared to other suburbs, where most people or a lot of people are Greek or Italian. They actually find pride in being wogs. They're not excluded because of it. I think that most people here have pride in their culture, whether they're Greek or Polish or Chinese or whatever.

There was a particular dress code associated with this group, which was more prescriptive than that for most other groups. It involved particular brands of sports wear and extreme hairstyles. Students in this group were heavy rather than experimental smokers, those with attitude, the ones who got into trouble with the teachers, and who felt victimised. They were not associated with academic success. Most of the 'wogs' at this school were born in Australia to parents born in Australia. However, the group was extended to include some immigrant students, most particularly some Russians. These Russians qualified as 'wogs' because of their migration experience and distinctly 'un-Australian' ways of being. In this regard, their link to Europe was also significant.

A school with a strict uniform code makes being a 'Goth' a strictly weekend affair. It was rumoured that Goths with their characteristic black clothing, pale complexions, and obvious makeup attended the school. However, their choice was witnessed on the rare occasions students were allowed to attend school in casual dress, commonly as a fund-raiser for charity. Students commented that a senior group of students were Goths and that a group had emerged at the junior level of the school as well. 'They just hang around together and act weird' was one Year 9 boy's description of this group. The Goths became a more significant marker in one staff member's mind. A group made the decision to leave the school 'Because they have to bend to the will of the school in terms of their appearance'. There was concern from this teacher that this gave students the message that individuality was not valued at Leafy Suburbs College.

Within the school community the named student subcultures had immense symbolic worth, yet with closer scrutiny, the labels encompassed so much difference that their worth became questionable. When asked to describe these terms, student interviewees, tended to fracture them into further categories. The 'wogs' for example, included the 'wanna be wogs' (those whose families had no history of migration); 'SOBs' (straight off the boat wogs) or those who were recent arrivals to Australia; and 'real wogs' (those whose parents or grandparents had migrated from Greece or Italy). As well as difference within the categories, there was also slippage between them. 'Asians' and 'nerds' were linked, as were 'popular' kids and 'musos'. While there was difference within and between these categories, the categories were far from benign. They also functioned to exclude. A recently arrived, chess-playing Russian could not be a 'wog' and was more likely to be accepted as a 'nerd'. On the other hand, a similar student who did not play chess but smoked instead was welcome within the 'wog' group. An 'Asian' violinist could not be a 'muso' and an athletic soccer player with Greek heritage couldn't be a 'jock'. So while being a 'jock' was linked to sport, it was also linked with traditional forms of Australian-ness and how these manifested through masculinities linked to Australian-rules football and cricket. The 'popular' kids were at the top of this particular food chain and while elite, this group was also eclectic. Membership was reserved for those who were good looking, fashionable, and of course 'cool'. It captured the best of the 'musos' and the 'jocks' but never any 'wogs' or 'Asians'. In this way, the categories were linked to real and imagined choices, which in turn were linked to embodiment. A 'wog', for example, could be a dark-haired Greek or a fair Russian, whereas being 'Asian-looking' allowed less room to move.

The 'hardcores' were described as hanging around at the back of the oval and smoking. This was a group associated with hip hop and rap music. They were seen as somewhat disengaged from the mainstream school culture, including academic achievement. Whilst smoking was not allowed at the school, students understood that the 'hardcores' (and the 'wogs') got away with it. At lunch time they chose to congregate under trees at the extreme edges of the school grounds.

By the time teachers reached them, the cigarettes had been butted out. Rather than escalate a cat-and-mouse chase, students described a form of appeasement that had developed. Some members of this group were also associated with the smoking of marijuana although this was understood to happen out of school.

Seeping and Silent Cultures

Implicit in the categories named above are a range of assumptions about gender and sexuality. In most cases the labels offered up as school subcultures did not differentiate between boys and girls. Yet when listening to the descriptions of such groups, it was easy to imagine that the descriptions given related to the most pronounced masculinities associated with such groups. Students described the 'wogs' who smoked on the oval and got into fights with the 'jocks' or 'hardcores'. In contradistinction to this, they described the nerds as playing chess, War Hammer, or four-square, all activities dominated by boys. There was no specific mention of how girls in such groups spent their time. The people named as characterising particular groups were most often boys. By implication, the girls offered similar and complimentary renditions of 'wog', 'nerd', 'Goth' etc. Their identities were linked to the group identity, which was defined by the boys. The exceptions to this pattern were the 'popular' and 'blonde' girls. Some students identified individual girls and linked them to a femininity that was 'bitchy', a term that had no male equivalent.

These subcultures assumed normative heterosexual relations. These were embedded in the association between 'jocks' and 'blonde' girls for example. The 'wog' category has been associated with strong forms of patriarchy linked to real, imagined, and constructed representations of machismo. 'Wog' girls were seen as tough and the boys as even tougher. The 'nerds' were assumed to have no social life, and thus also assumed to have no sexual life. Implicit in determinations of what constituted 'popular' was appealing to members of the opposite sex. However, while normative heterosexual relations were the benchmark, there was a group of openly homosexual and bisexual male students at the school. They were happy to be identified as gay and talked openly about this issue. A very popular teacher was openly homosexual. The school seemed to provide a clear message of inclusion around this issue for staff and students. The staff list provided for this research by the Principal indicated that there were two same-sex couples on staff, although gender was not specified. A number of homosexual and bisexual boys were involved in the music and theatre programs and in this context were respected for their talent, openness, and joie de vivre. It was clear to some of these students, however, that this type of involvement was somewhat of a cliché and this created feelings of ambivalence for them. One openly gay boy described what he felt was a teacher's over acceptance of him and how he found this 'patronising'. During the course of this study, no one spoke as a lesbian or about lesbianism.

Some students at the school were Jewish. Other students described them as not 'seriously' Jewish because they attended a Government school rather than an Independent Jewish school. One teacher argued that at the school 'it's just *really* normal to be Jewish, you're just *not* discriminated against at all.' In Australia, the Jewish community encompasses a range of difference in terms of place of origin, length of Australian residency, and levels of religious orthodoxy. This was reflected at Leafy Suburbs College where some Jewish students were born in Russia, South Africa, and Israel and others had families that had been in Australia for many generations. A Jewish youth organisation functioned at the school. In this sense, the Jewish presence was obvious, but as a subculture amongst the students, it was not obvious. Knowing whether a 'nerd', 'muso' or 'popular kid' was Jewish was seen as irrelevant. One Jewish student described it as follows:

> I think it's like an underlying thing, like all the Jewish people know who they are and like everyone knows who you are and stuff if you're Jewish, but I don't think it's one of the main aspects which determines your social group.

Student drug and alcohol consumption is an issue that captures the public imagination. As a consequence, providing a drug-free environment has become a marker for a 'good' school. A good school is one where students do not take drugs and there has been an association between laxity on this issue and Government schools. Independent schools relative to Government schools are able to police entry of students and expel students more readily and this is judged to provide them with more control over drug taking within their communities. In Victoria, there had been debate amongst such schools as to the benefits of compulsory drug testing of students. Would such a move breach individual rights, help eradicate drug use, or simply signal to parents (clients) that the school takes a hard line on the matter? Leafy Suburbs College was understood to take an unforgiving position on drugs. Immediate expulsion would result regardless of type of drug and amount. On one occasion, police were summoned to escort two boys off the school premises because they had been caught with what was understood by students to be a small amount of cannabis. The Principal immediately called a whole-school assembly to explain what had happened and reiterated the school policy on drugs. Students spoke of seeing their peers in the back of a police car and seeing the emotional impact this decision had had on the Principal and staff at the school. Nonetheless, students at the school did take drugs. One mother described how her son smoked marijuana and how this was interfering with his academic progress. She described how he often stayed home to smoke with a neighbour. During the course of the study, this boy was expelled from Leafy

Suburbs College. Other students spoke of senior and respected 'musos' who smoked marijuana. In this way, students distinguished between 'stoners' whose life seemed out of control and those who they saw as involved in more benign forms of recreational drug taking.

> You can picture the kids that come in Year 7 that are going to be one of the exit ones at Year 10. They aren't particularly academic and don't particularly want to try, and don't have a habit, or don't perhaps have expectations from family, that they will put in the discipline that's needed. I would guess there are probably about twenty kids who would leave the school at about Year 10 or 11 looking for alternatives to what we offer.

The above comment was made by a member of staff. Perhaps the most silent culture at the school was that related to failure. Parents, education professionals, and teachers, including those not directly associated with the school, spoke about the rigorous academic demands placed on students at Leafy Suburbs College. In this context, while enrolment was sought after, there was also an understanding that the environment did not suit all students. In a school where demand outstrips supply, enrolment is constructed as more a privilege than a right. In this climate, there is less incentive and opportunity to reflect on the advantages of providing a school culture that is inclusive of a broader range of students. Instead, students who did not fit into the culture of the school were counselled (more or less aggressively) to leave. This was understood as good for these students because their sense of failure would be ameliorated at another school where it was presumed they would be happier. Additionally, some teachers described this as fairer because it allowed students, better suited to the school culture and 'waiting on the doorstep', access to a much sought-after resource currently being wasted. These understandings were commonly linked to students' study habits and willingness to try rather than to notions of innate academic ability. In this sense, students' nonconformity was constructed as personal choice. These nonconforming students were counselled about their academic endeavours. This counselling was particularly virulent at the end of Year 10 but could begin earlier. Amongst the students, there were common-sense understandings that students who failed would not be tolerated and asked to leave. Year-level coordinators took responsibility for academic progress and linked to this, discipline and welfare. This nexus between discipline, welfare, and academic progress arguably represents the engine room of schooling at Leafy Suburbs College. In students' minds, the school was good because it 'forced' them to work harder, which they believed was for their own benefit. Yet they also believed the school was too strict, inflexible, and unforgiving. In this sense, those who failed to conform were counselled to leave the school. However, conformity was fluid and responsive primarily to academic achievement. A student who attained good academic results was forgiven a more creative interpretation of the uniform code, for example. A student who was understood as a 'bad' academic investment could be hounded for minor breaches of the uniform code. Individual coordinators varied in their approach to academic progress, discipline, and welfare. Their interpretation and implementation of guidelines was responsive to their own philosophy and priorities. Some were more generous and flexible, reading between the lines of students' behaviour, their intentions, their circumstances, and their strengths and weaknesses. Others presented a narrow interpretation of what was possible. In general, staff interviewed supported the strong discipline at the school and argued that it contributed to the high academic standards. However, some coordinators and teachers were critical of their peers for being overly rigid in their implementation of discipline at the school.

Eagleton (2000) makes the point that culture is not inherently political and that instead it becomes so only if it is caught up within dynamics of domination and resistance. Leafy Suburbs College is a school that is caught up in the dynamics of domination and resistance that are produced by market forces. It represents a paradox in that it is one of very few Government schools in suburban Melbourne that goes close to providing students with scores that facilitate entry into university, particularly elite universities. In some ways this paradox represents an act of resistance against what Teese and Polesel (2003) describe as the stability of the hierarchy that characterises educational achievement. However, this resistance is achieved through the provision of an arguably narrow rendition of academic culture. In itself, this academic culture is experienced as oppressive by various groups of students who for different reasons find themselves excluded. In a school where there is little room to accommodate various definitions of success, how do students from different subcultures mediate the dominant school culture in relation to their own imagined futures? In the chapters to follow, this question is explored through interviews with students who were, at least initially, associated with some of the subcultures identified here.

Chapter 6

Being In 'Geek Kingdom'

A major aim of this book is to consider how student identities, school cultures, and imagined futures interrelate at a school like Leafy Suburbs College, where traditional understandings of academic success are interpreted by groups of students for whom such success is not always assumed. Students interviewed identified particular subcultures and linked each with specific attributes. There existed shared understandings amongst students (and some teachers) as to these groups, their names, and the attributes associated with each. However, once this landscape was sketched, individual students were reluctant to place themselves into these subcultures. Many could see why others had identified them with a particular group, but did not want to own the label. It was not possible to interview students from all the subcultures identified as existing within the school. To this extent, the identification of some subcultures as 'silent', tells as much of a story about my capacity to make visible or bring to voice particular groups of students as it does about the students and the school. However, being more or less 'interviewable', therefore, counts for something and I'm hesitant to dismiss as coincidence the fact that the groups easiest to interview were those associated with subcultures with relatively high standing amongst students. In this sense, the interpretation of how school subcultures operate offered by the most 'interviewable', needs to be contextualised in relation to their place in the school. In this way, the exploration offered here has been framed by the worldview of those students with a particular kudos. The kudos is worth considering at two levels. First, it is linked to students' standing within the school community. Second, it is also linked to the research dynamic itself. Some groups were easier to access and some groups found it easier to access the research intention. In other words, interviewees spoke 'research' with various levels of fluency. Because of this, some students' experiences were more or less opaque to me than those of others.

In this chapter, an interview with four Year 10 students will be explored in depth. This was the first interview with students undertaken and as such it is significant in shaping my initial view of how subcultures were constituted at the school. Further to this, it became somewhat of a benchmark for how an interview should and could operate. With hindsight it has become clear that this interview provided unrealistic expectations that would frame subsequent interviews negatively by comparison. This group of four students was exceptionally fluent at speaking 'research'. Had I not interviewed them first, others would have seemed more articulate. However, interviews were arranged when and with whom was possible at any given time and the first of anything is likely to have disproportionate impact. These students were academically successful. Their comments provide particularly productive insights because of this; that is, they functioned successfully within the school but were nonetheless critical about many of its features. Most specifically, I am interested here to consider how these students described the school subcultures, their places within these, the possibility of shifting between such subcultures, and the relationships of the subcultures to their imagined futures.

Stephen, an 'Asian-looking' boy, was in the accelerated learning program. He was openly gay and central to the school theatre program. Miread, an 'Australian' girl, was planning to leave the school at the end of the year. Daniel had parents born overseas in different countries and avoided naming his ethnic heritage. He and Paul, who was 'Australian', were both heavily involved in the music program. These four students had been friends since beginning at Leafy Suburbs College. Paul and Stephen had attended the same primary school as well. These students considered themselves as friends and had an easy rapport with each other. They had in common their love of learning and wish to succeed academically. While these students were happy to describe the general school population through the subcultures described in the previous chapter, they were reluctant to identify personally with any one of them. When asked to comment on this discrepancy, they argued that such labels had decreasing relevancy as students matured. These markers were most significant between Years 7 and 9. They had been identified with a number of these subcultures when they were younger. Miread, for example, had been a 'blonde' girl and she was quick to defend this group against the stereotypes of them as 'stupid and bitchy'. Daniel and Paul had slipped in and out of being 'nerds' and 'musos'. While for Stephen the major identity issue centred on his sexuality, the decision and consequences of coming out as gay. He felt that others would see him as a 'nerd'. The interview was conducted near the end of the school year when Year 10 students were being counselled by VCE coordinators. This was a rigorous process during which students were individually interviewed and on the basis of Year 10 results guided into Year 11 and 12 subjects. Some students, seen as less well suited to the academic program offered at the school, were advised to seek enrolment at neighbourhood schools with more flexible curricula. The group interview began thus:

GT: Ok, what type of students do you think succeed in the school here?

Miread: Depends, do you mean succeed academically?

GT: Well, that's open for debate.

Miread: Um ... people who fit the system.

GT: You mean academically?

Miread: Yeah.

Paul: What type of groups are we talking about? Are we talking about ethnic groups or are we talking about geeks? Because honestly the people who achieve at Leafy Suburbs College are the geeks!

Stephen: What's your definition of a geek?

Paul: I don't know! But the geeks achieve!

GT: I'm really interested. What's a geek?

Paul: I don't know, it's just the people who, oh shit I'm kind of labelling myself here. They're kind of the people who just bury themselves in books because they enjoy the books! 'Geek' is a term that no longer can be used as derogatory.

Stephen: I think it's an American television thing that they used in the nineties to degrade people. You had the 'geeks', you had the 'losers' and you had the 'jocks' and the 'cheerleaders'.

GT: Yeah, but what is a geek?

Miread: Not very good socially.

Daniel: They usually failed socially and made up for that by being academic.

Paul: But now it's changing and the majority of people at Leafy Suburbs College in the older levels are the geeks.

Stephen: You can be smart.

Paul:	But they're still social because there are so many geeks! They're all relating to each other! There's this 'geek kingdom' here, that kind of reaches out to all the geeks!
Stephen:	It's just changed from probably in the seventies and stuff where people didn't have to do heaps of work and you just came to school to talk to your friends and go out on the weekends and party hard. They've just changed so much.
GT:	You mean my age group?
Stephen:	Yeah! It's just changed so much that in modern days, you want to achieve and you work hard but you also have a fun time while doing it. So geeks don't really exist anymore because lots of people are doing school work and they are smart but they also have a life.
Daniel:	I don't think that line exists between social failures who do well and the social successors who do badly. In my experience and I haven't been anywhere else.

These students confirmed the stereotype of the 'geek' and in almost the same breath, denied it existed. Their immediate response was to create a dichotomy between the academic and the social, understanding these as mutually exclusive. Yet they also constructed this stereotype as one created through the media with more relevance to a bygone era. Importantly, it was a stereotype that their own identities dismantled.

GT:	So are you kids geeks?
Miread:	In a way.
Stephen:	Yeah, I would be considered one.
Paul:	Yeah.
Miread:	I'm like a humanities geek, and I'm really passionate about what I like, and I love reading. I get into a book and I'm up the whole night, and I'm into my music — I'm obsessive about all of that. So if you call that geeky then I don't care but I'm really social so I don't have any social problems. I don't think and I don't you know — so I s'pose I'm not really because I'm not that academic.
Daniel:	Yeah, like I said before I don't think there's that line anymore.
Paul:	Yeah, but some people still see the line. Some of the people in our year still see it.
Daniel:	Of course, you still have those kids who are absolute jocks and the kids who are walking calculators, but they're a very small minority.
Paul:	But even the small minority — the rest of us will talk to them, the rest of us aren't afraid of the two extremes and we'll still speak to them. Like I hang

out with the hardcore geeks at lunchtime and stuff and they're a great bunch to be around.

Stephen had less ambivalence about his status as a 'geek'. In this group, he was the only student in the accelerated learning program. Miread broadens this definition of 'geek' by describing herself as a 'humanities geek' and then qualifies her comment by noting her social capabilities. 'I'm not that academic' belies her struggle to be both 'geek' and socially competent. Daniel argues against the division and at the same time confirms it through his reference to 'jocks' and 'walking calculators'. By posing the extremes, he opens the possibility for a space in-between, one I suspect he is most comfortable to occupy. Paul confirms these extremes and positions himself in the 'majority', but nonetheless, happy to socialise with 'hardcore geeks'. Paul has insights into this because he plays cards at lunchtime and this activity draws together a disparate group of students.

Daniel: That card game that you play is like the mixing of the two extremes.

Stephen: I've got no idea what that type of character is.

GT: Card game?

Paul: I play cards at lunchtime.

Stephen: See, you guys tend to mix the normal guys with the nerds. So you've got Robert the geek and the other Robert the stoner.

Paul: He's not a stoner! He's only a little bit of a stoner!

GT: And a stoner is someone who smokes pot?

Paul: He's not a stoner he's just tasted it once … or twice!

Through cards we have another element introduced. Along with the 'geeks' and the 'normal guys' we have the 'stoner', someone who has experimented with cannabis. Stephen was the first to introduce the 'jocks' and 'popular chicks' into the conversation and he positioned these students at one end of a spectrum. These were the students who had the power to make other students feel 'like shit'.

Jocks and Blondes

Stephen: So like Daniel said, you've still got the extremes like the jocks and the popular chicks, who sit round doing nothing. They usually think they're at the top but most people don't like them. But for some reason they hold power that they don't have. They're the bullies of the school, they make people feel like shit and they have people follow them.

Paul: Miread's got her finger in the power point — the proverbial power point. She's friends with all the popular girls.

Stephen: Yeah, but she's a normal person.

Miread: So people say to me, 'Oh those girls, they think they're so good they just sit there thinking they're so good. And they just sit there talking about … a tree or something'. People make them out to be so stupid and so …

GT: Describe them for me …

Miread: It depends on where you see them from … because people assume that they're these evil bitchy girls that are just so horrible.

Daniel: Like the whole blonde cheerleader group.

Miread: But, really, they're … I've been in other groups of girls that say 'Oh we're not like them, they're so bitchy' and then they bitch about each other. And this group, they all like each other and they barely ever fight and they're quite happy with themselves and then these other groups say, 'They're so bitchy', and then they're all backstabbing.

Stephen: It's because this group makes other people feel like shit.

Paul: When she's [Miread] talking about bitching groups that are bitching about the groups that are supposedly bitching. Well, the friends that I made this year and last year I probably won't be friends with any longer because the key person that I was great friends with … I was great friends with her and so I was great friends with all her friends. But … she's leaving and I don't want to hang out with these people because they do not shut up about how much a pain in the arse each one of them are. It just drives me nuts!

Daniel: I think it's a girl thing.

Miread: Yeah, it is, because I'm not into the whole bitching rah rah rah, because I can't get along with girls … like, the people who say that they're lower than them are often meaner to these girls. Like the popular girls cop a lot of crap because they're blonde and a lot of people are really jealous of them and I feel sorry for them because a few of the girls are pretty genuine people and they cop all this stuff and everybody assumes that they must be these bimbos, and everyone stereotypes them.

Daniel: You asked where the power came from, and I think it comes from the fact that there are some people who are very secure and happy with themselves and there are people outside that sphere who are a lot less secure and insecure, I s'pose and jealous.

Paul: And they bag other people who are secure making them insecure and then … (laughs)

During the interview, Miread was positioned as both a 'popular' girl and 'normal'. She had insights into this group because she had been a member. She expressed her loyalty to the group of girls who people assumed were 'bitchy' and characterised as 'bimbos'. She argued that these girls suffered the consequences of the stereotype but in reality they were good friends and 'pretty genuine'. There was a feeling that their status made others jealous of them. Stephen, on the other hand, was more interested in the power these groups exerted.

> Yeah, but back to the people who have the power ... I'm going to use Lisa and Sarina as an example — they are quite self-obsessed people and they have the support of all the jock guys and they have double standards and they make other people feel like crap. And you watch any high school TV show and — I know TVs not real blah blah blah — but you find that there's always a group who are the hierarchy that most people don't like but fear them because they hold the power. They make fun of people. I remember this incident, it was in Year 8 or something — it's quite lame but. At our school canteen there's always a big thing about pushing and shoving because the canteen's so slow and I was next to those two girls and they decided it was OK to shove me over, and I wasn't going to take that crap from them so I shoved her back. And because of their double standards, the fact that they think they're in a higher position than me because of my social standing and the fact that they're top shit — no one should be able to push them — they didn't like that and so they told all their guy friends and I copped shit like 'Hey what are you doing pushing them'. (Stephen)

While Stephen considered the incident in the canteen as 'lame' or trivial, it was also an exemplar in his mind of the lived experience of hierarchy at the school. He was aware of his 'social standing' relative to that of the popular girls and his vulnerability at the hands of the 'jocks' who were their 'guy friends'. In this way the 'blonde' girls represented a complex set of heterosexual relationships and the unequal power relations that underpin these. Daniel's comment that 'it's a girl thing' and Miread's defence of these girls against the stereotype of the blonde bimbo illustrate both the benefit and the cost of this power for girls seen as conforming to dominant enactments of sexuality. Paul's feeling of nonbelonging given the departure of the 'popular' girl who was his friend within this group illustrates how a boy who does not immediately present as a 'jock' has another set of issues with which to deal. The 'blonde' girls whose cause was being championed by the 'jocks' illustrated the unequal power relations that immediately positioned some students on the periphery, acutely aware of 'double standards' enacted as bullying. Dominant forms of heterosexuality position students differentially and it is not surprising that this issue was upper most in Stephen's mind given his 'social standing' as homosexual, 'geek' and 'Asian' looking. In this context, Miread's worth was elevated because she had chosen to forgo her membership of the 'popular chicks'. Clearly the choice of being both 'popular' and 'normal' could be open only to those already deemed popular.

GT: Are they really blonde?

Miread:	That's what annoys me! They are actually pretty blonde, but like, people used to say to me, 'Oh you're a part of the blonde group' and I'd be like 'Look at my hair! It's brown!' It's just stupid.
Paul:	No, it's the blonde stereotype. The blonde label doesn't always mean the blonde hair, but because of all the blonde jokes it just means the ditzy chicks.
GT:	And the jocks — tell me more.
Paul:	Well, the jocks have been changing now; they used to just be the group that excelled at sport and sat in class drooling, but now it's changed and …
GT:	But are they sort of, an inner group?
Paul:	Yeah, but a lot of the people that I would consider idiots and jocks, like I've become friends with a couple of them like Gary. Gary's into football and cricket and rugby and he loves it but he's pulling A's and A+'s in every single class. Like I can have these amazing conversations with him but looking at him you think 'Oh geez pass the football'.
Daniel:	And he does have a very 'ocker' way of speaking. He's very 'G'day mate'.
Stephen:	I always associate the jocks with not just sport; you say it's changing, people who are good at sport or good at academics don't come under jocks in my books. The jock category are the guys who are quite stupid, they are rude and immature, and they make fun of people who are weaker than them, they are bullies, they make other people feel bad, and they're normally good at sport and friends with the popular girls.
Paul:	The jocks that I'm thinking of, not going to mention names but Liam [whispers] he's …
Stephen:	An idiot!
Paul:	No, he wouldn't be classed as a jock, but he's been doing Tae Kwon Do for 12 years, so he's been doing it since he was like 5, and he's an amazingly fit guy, but you could hit him in the head and he wouldn't lose a brain cell, mainly because he doesn't have any to lose!
Stephen:	Stupid! But he lit firecrackers at school! Yeah, that was just so stupid.
Daniel:	Outside the staffroom.
Stephen:	And the Year 12 coordinator walked past.
Daniel:	With the teacher just there.

Implied but never stated was the link between these students and their ethnic background. The link between the 'jocks' and a form of Australian masculinity made famous by Paul Hogan was hinted at through the reference to 'footy', being 'ocker' and saying 'g'day'. Yet these students were clear that being 'blonde' had no ethnic derivation. It is most common for 'ethnic' to be associated with minorities rather than the majority and in Australia being 'ethnic' implies having a background associated with migration (Castles et al. 1988; Tsolidis 2001; Hage 2003). By the end of this conversation there seemed to be less rather than more consensus about 'blondes' and 'jocks'. Jocks could be intelligent and blondes did not have to be blonde. Only Stephen remained unswerving in his definition. 'Jocks' were not academic, usually played sport, and most importantly, they were characterised by their friendship with 'popular' girls and their bullying of other students. In Stephen's mind, this type of popularity was associated with the power that allowed some students to make other students feel bad about themselves.

Homophobic Bullying

Stephen, Miread, Paul, and Daniel did not openly identify themselves with any one subculture and instead stressed the possibilities of moving between them. Daniel played cricket with the 'jocks', Paul was a 'band geek' because of his heavy involvement in the music program. Miread stated, 'I'm sort of everywhere, I'm not really in a group. I'm just a bit of everything'. Describing the ease most students felt operating between groups, Paul drew attention to homophobia.

Paul: We all can talk to each other. Except maybe Stephen with the homophobes, because they wouldn't like you.

GT: And are they a big group in the school?

Stephen: Ummm ... Leafy Suburbs College is actually quite good with a lot of accepting people, but there are still a lot of pricks at the school.

Paul: They just want to be pricks.

Miread: They're just scared, and they don't understand it. Maybe it's just their upbringing, they just aren't introduced, well you can't really tell.

GT: And is there a gay group at the school?

Stephen: Not really ... I don't think so.

Paul: I don't think so. I don't think there's enough in the school.

Stephen: There's not enough open people in the school to have a certain group because as far as I know there's two in Year 12 — this year's Year 12. There's one or two in Year 11 and two in Year 10 and I know of at least one in Year 9 and they're all different people.

Daniel: Like they're totally different, like Stephen's probably one of my best mates but then you've got this other guy who is so annoying!

Paul:	It's not his sexuality, it's his personality. Honestly I'm not quite sure if he's gay or not, I asked him one time why he chose to be gay and he's gone, 'It's more out there than being bisexual' and I said, 'Well, then, why are you bisexual?' And he said, 'It's more interesting than being straight'. So I'm not actually sure if he actually is gay or seeks the attention.
Daniel:	He's a big kid, and I don't think many people would pay much attention if he wasn't gay.
Stephen:	He's quite a fake person as well … the way he acts and the way he moves. You look at him and think that it's not genuine you would think he's faking it for attention. Where as me and others, we're genuine people.
GT:	But do you feel harassed?
Stephen:	Oh, harassed constantly. More so now than before. It's getting to me more now than it used to.
GT:	What's changed?
Paul:	I couldn't believe that George guy … that freaked me out. Well, weren't you two good mates and then he found out and he dropped you like a sack of potatoes?
Stephen:	He didn't drop me. He was the first person I told because he was my best mate, but he didn't drop me as such, he just became really rude and treated me like shit and our relationship fell apart.
Daniel:	Also, we had a group in Year 7. Year 7 is groups. It's just groups, there's a group here and a group here, and they all stand in little pods around the school. Whereas now, it sort of blends out a bit. Problem being — you're [directed at Stephen] not in any of my classes, and I think if you were in my classes, you would get harassed less because you're with us.
Stephen:	I'd have more support … because in …
Daniel:	See they split us up though and we can't do anything about who's in each class.
Stephen:	Yeah, because I had English where I'm practically alone, and I've got arseholes like Sam and Tom and Lenny and … you just have to deal with them. You can't really stop it.
Miread:	These are like the good-looking, think-they're-god's-gift-to-women guys, they walk around, they're just disgusting. They think they're just so high up and you're just like — ' get real'.
Paul:	Some of them are all right when you get to know them. I don't know Sam, but I know Lenny …
Stephen:	You don't want to.

During this discussion Stephen made it obvious that the support that meant the most to him came from his friendship group, students like Daniel and Miread who had been with him since at least Year 7. He stated that he did not speak about his sexuality with staff, including those who were openly gay. Instead, he had developed a range of understandings about how bullying worked, the attitudes that caused it, and how the system failed to prevent such behaviour.

Stephen: See, that's where bullies become smart. They pick opportunities where teachers can't do anything. Whether it's just little bumps in the corridor or passing comments.

Daniel: Like he never gets bagged when he's around us, like around me and Miread it won't happen.

Stephen: It's only when I'm by myself … that's because the people are weak, maybe they don't really believe in what they're making out they believe in. They're just thinking ' Oh let's just have a little fun'. So when I'm around friends, they wouldn't dare.

Miread: Hmm … yeah definitely.

Stephen: Also because I've spread myself out through the school, I've got friends in Year 9 and friends in Year 10, and I've got a lot of friends in Year 11, that's also caused me to cop a bit more shit, because I've been harassed by people in Year 11 which is a bit tough. You have to try and get over it; it's part of the world and it's always going to happen. And it's going to take centuries for it to go away, if, in fact, it ever does. You just have to stay strong.

Relative to the others, Stephen had the most acute sense of how power operated having experienced its excesses more than the other three. His strongest sense of support grew from the relationships he had developed with the students who had known him for a long time and appreciated him for his 'genuine' self. During this short exchange, I was struck by how someone his age had developed a strength and stoicism and yet I was left depressed by how he seemed to carry this burden with little institutional support. These students dismissed as not worthwhile the system of support available through the school's welfare structures. Rightly or wrongly, they understood these as incapable of guaranteeing confidentiality and of only supplying well-meaning but ineffectual caring. They described the Welfare Officer as the extreme opposite to the Deputy Principal, who they saw as a harsh disciplinarian. Nonetheless, they caricatured the Welfare Officer in the following way:

Paul: 'Let's drink herbal tea!'

Stephen: 'Hi! I'll be your friend!'

Daniel: Send you a letter every week asking how you're going, and sort of gets up your nose about how much can I help you.

Silenced Cultures

During the interview, these students reminded me that I needed to speak with students who weren't like them. Miread seemed the most sensitive to the needs of the students who she understood as on the periphery of the dominant school culture. Given her decision to leave the school, this did not seem surprising. She saw the school as excluding her brother who was not a traditional academic performer and at various points in the interview seemed to advocate on behalf of such students. She did not offer a comment on the welfare structures at the school, seeming more content to say nothing rather than join the negative banter about this type of caring. She struck me as an extraordinary girl, someone with quiet confidence and an ability to cut to the core of any issue but remain empathetic. The following sequence provides some illustration of this.

Miread:	Something that we didn't talk about is something about students that succeed. You know how there's always going to be people that get into drugs and stuff, there's a big group of people that are into that sort of stuff, and they generally — don't succeed.
Paul:	Don't succeed …
Miread:	They … they, a lot of them have dropped out and a lot of them are in trouble with the school, they're …
Stephen:	They won't let the teacher's help them …
Daniel:	Also, I'm going to take the example of Patrick. He's really amazingly talented …
Stephen:	Stoner
Daniel:	But he's really smart, and he's really … I think he wants to be a teacher and I would have no problems with him teaching my kids, but he's on drugs and the school doesn't want to know him because of it.
Miread:	He actually has real problems in his head with drugs … he's pretty much been doing it since primary school, because I went to primary school with him.
Paul:	The only stuff he didn't do was heroin because his brother OD-ed on it.
Daniel:	His brother was really bad.
GT:	How do they get the money for it?
Stephen:	Borrow money, out of mum's purse.
Miread:	And the thing is, the problem is his parents smoke weed.
Paul:	Yeah, they were the original problem …
Miread:	Yeah, so he's been brought up on it … so he'll say to his mum 'Oh, mum, I want a gram of it, I'm getting stoned tonight', she'll say, 'Oh, ok'.

Paul:	But he can still function, he can write these amazing stories, he's an amazing literature kid ... he can still function on it.
Miread:	But he does have mental problems ... that's the thing. I said to him, 'So why don't you just stop for Year 12?' 'Oh, because weed's there, when no one else is', and just stuff like that. He's got a couple of problems. Yeah, so I think that drugs really affect your achievement.

Miread's concerns about this student seemed to congeal around three issues: his need for support because of his 'mental problems', the fact that she understood these problems stemming from bad parenting, and the school's seeming inability to offer such a student an alternative way forward. Instead, he was left to make his own way through what life had meted out to him, using drugs as a prop and wasting what Miread understood as obvious aptitude.

As an interviewer, you need to be aware of the fine line between pushing forward relentlessly and having an interview finish without engagement with one of your 'favourite topics'. These students silenced the issue of ethnic difference. As the interview drew to a close, I made the decision to raise it rather than foreclose on the possibility of some comment. They were very forthcoming in their response, which leaves me with the task of reading their initial silence as a type of disengagement with the topic or a type of nervousness prompted by who I am (an overtly 'ethnic' interviewer) and the connotations of appearing to highlight ethnic issues in this context. Interviews are complex interactions, and who we are and how we see each other overlay them. Whilst two of these students had minority backgrounds, they did not foreground this aspect of their identities until this point of the interview. Perhaps my prompt and how I am embodied as 'ethnic' could be read as either silencing or providing permission to speak on a topic that can be divisive.

GT:	One of the things no one's talked about is the ethnic stuff ... is that an issue?
Paul:	Um ... not really. You have a little chuckle at those totally Orthodox Jews that come around and wait after school for certain kids and you have a little chuckle because it's 35°C and they're wearing like full black clothes and ...
Daniel:	Oh, they're the ones that hand out pamphlets and stuff.
Stephen:	And they're all like preachy ... and you're like 'Get away, don't be preachy, I'll do what I want'.
Daniel:	Seriously, I'm half Jewish.
Stephen:	Me too.
Daniel:	And they were standing out the front of the school handing out forms and trying to get people interested and the thing was, and they asked me if I was

Jewish and I said, 'Well, I'm sort of Jewish, does that count?' Because it's sort of a long story, because in the Middle East they're chauvinist bastards and my dad's side is from there, so the Jewish goes down the father's side, whereas here it goes down the mother's side. So here I'm not Jewish, there [Middle East] I am. And he didn't want to know me. I was just interested to see how they'd react and ... they didn't want to know me. See, those people stand out the front of the school in their full dress and they'd probably never get bashed up or insulted because of the Jewish locals ... and people will walk past and say, 'Oh, did you see that?' But the good thing is, they'll never get it outside.

Stephen: I think it's so annoying with how preachy they are. I actually went home another way just because I didn't want to be preached by them, because I'd spoken to a friend and ...

Paul: Just kiss one of them and they'd never talk to you again ... [everyone laughs]

Stephen: Yeah ... [laughs], it's just they're kind of annoying and it's with most religions. I just don't think its appropriate being outside our school being preachy with religion.

Miread: Um ... no, I think they have a right to educate us.

Paul: But the way they do it is wrong.

Daniel: Basically, they try to convert us without being rash. They're trying to find the Jews who are like me, but full Jewish and dress normally and don't do everything Jewish and they're trying to convert us.

Stephen: They're trying to turn us into them ... and you're just like, 'Get lost, I don't want big side burns and funny hats and things coming off my belt!'

The first response to my question on 'ethnic stuff' comes from Paul who would be identified as 'real' Australian. He speaks about a group that is distinct in terms of appearance and interaction with the school community. Prior to this point, I was unaware of the religious affiliation of these students and remain unaware whether Paul knew of Stephen and Daniel's status as 'half Jewish'. Daniel's comment that the Jewish 'locals' make overt signs of Jewishness less risky, hints at experiences of anti-Semitism. Stephen refuses to be confronted by the group at the front gate altogether and the 'preachy' aspect, rather than the Jewishness is something he wants to avoid. His homosexuality and its assumed status within an orthodoxy is taken up by Paul. The flippant comment that a kiss would liberate him from their attention is received light-heartedly and his statement that 'They're trying to turn us into them' sums up his desire to remain 'genuine', that is, true to his core identity. Nonetheless, it is the overt aspects of appearance he rejects most vehemently. Relative to the Daniel and Stephen who understand that they are the targets of such activity, Paul and Miread discuss the matter in relation to process and the 'right to educate us'. Miread is the first to move the discussion away from religion.

Miread: Well, I think, not with religion, but with actual background and race, there's a lot of groups. There's a lot of Russians and they have their own group, they all speak Russian and I understand they all like to speak to each other in Russian.

GT: Are they new arrivals?

Miread: Yeah.

Daniel: Yeah, so that's obvious ... and they're going to keep separate and speak Russian.

Paul: The guys who achieve a lot are the Asians. They achieve a lot more than any of us ... because this is the academic school. They come over here and do the advanced maths methods and the specialist maths and stuff and it's the stuff they've been doing in Grade 2, and they get like 97 and stuff.

Stephen: It's 'cause they're brought up in Japan and stuff, because they're brought up there they do an outstanding amount of work at school. They get made to do lots of homework from a young age, so I just think in countries like that they have a better work ethic, than we do. So when they come here they achieve really high because they're just used to it.

GT: And are they new arrivals too?

Paul: Less.

Daniel: Sometimes they're not. Their parents are always born over there.

Miread: And a lot of the time their parents couldn't succeed because they didn't have the facilities and the school and everything, so they put it through their kid to achieve. Like they want them to achieve because they couldn't sort of.

The newly arrived Russians are ethnicised, but this is a response to their status as new arrivals. They share each other's company because of their facility with Russian relative to English. However, in their few comments about 'Asians' these students confirm the dominant discourses about their association with academic achievement, a severe work ethic, and a hunger for achievement promulgated by parents with fewer opportunities. Similarly, the emphasis on mathematics in their countries of origin and how this advantages them in Australia is a common understanding. These students, however, seem unaware of the details of origin and birthplace. Being 'Asian' and 'brought up in Japan' stands in for detailed knowledge of actual ethnicity. Indeed, only six students at the school had a connection with Japan. It is understandable that students would identify ethnicity with the most overt forms of difference, in this case,

Orthodox Jews, 'Asians' and newly arrived Russians. Still, there is a silence about the 'wogs', a category the same interviewees identified when nominating the subcultures in the school more generally. Again, I prompt a response, in part recognising that in these terms, I would be associated with the 'wogs' and that perhaps these students need more permission to speak on this issue than on some of the others.

Wogs — 'It's Like a Sovereign State'

GT: And what about wogs?

Paul: Who?

GT: The groups that are called wogs?

Daniel: They're proud of it ... they're so proud of it!

GT: They're here too? Do they do well? Are they jocks or musos or ...

Paul: They come as ... they don't do very well.

Stephen: The wogs are usually kind of ...

Daniel: There's this one Alex Stefanov ... comes in with his big stereo on his shoulder.

Paul: He's like 5 foot 3, he's this tiny little guy.

Daniel: But he's so full of himself.

GT: Where is he from?

Paul: I don't know ... I think he's Russian, but he wants to be ...

Miread: There's a lot of ... especially with the girls, they're born in Australia, they speak with no accent, and then they get to Year 9 and they think, 'Hey being a wog is cool'.

Paul: Well, suddenly we can speak weird! [mimicking the wog accent].

Miread: And they develop these accents ... it's funny!

Daniel: 'Wog' can't be called a derogatory sound at all any more ... it's like a status ...

Miread: They love it so much.

GT: Why?

Miread: Because they think that ...

Stephen: It makes them different and interesting.

Daniel: It's very arrogant though.

GT: So how would you characterise? Because you don't link these groups with academic achievement, no?

Daniel: No ... it's a social thing because they develop the accent, they get the friends, they start to dress differently, they smoke, the wog thing is a total ...

Paul: They get really pushy, they want to start a fight with anyone they can find.

GT: And they don't hang around with anyone else?

Paul: Nah, just the wogs.

Stephen: You tend not to take any notice anymore. You just do your own thing and don't give a shit what other people do.

Miread: Like a lot of them I used to be friends with, but now they see themselves as higher than me because they're big, big wog chicks and they've got all their wog boys, and why would you want an Aussie chick ... and a lot of the time 'Aussie' is used derogatively. They're like ... 'Oh, you must have a European background ...' and I'd say, 'Nah, nah, I'm totally Australian' and they're like 'Oh!'

Daniel: But it's different, like, it's a separate hierarchy. Even the most popular cheerleader will still be nothing but dirt and divided from the wogs. It's like a separate hierarchy.

Paul: It's like a sovereign state.

Daniel: It's like this smokers' corner in the back of the oval.

Paul: Well, there's two. I hang around with a lot of the smokers. I don't smoke myself because it's like a throw-your-life-away-on-a-stick-of-cancer, but you know, we can't sit down there anymore because they cut down the trees so there's nowhere to hide. But when we used to sit down there, there was all these, the Australians come down this side, and the wogs would be on the other side ... and we started this war, because we took one of their seats! It was great ... because they've got all these park benches on the oval, we took one of them and put it on our side and they were like 'We want you guys to bring it back over here now' [wog accent] and we were like 'Nah, we're not going to ...' so they poured honey all over it ... it was great. They wouldn't take it back over there themselves.

Daniel: I think there's only been one fight the whole time I've been here.

Miread: I've seen about four.

Daniel: Thompson and Johnno. He was the biggest guy — Thompson — in primary school, when I played cricket with him, he seemed like a nice guy.

Miread: He is such a horrible guy.

Daniel: He seemed nice, but everyone tells me that he's evil.

Paul: He went to my primary school and he was always the bully, and nothing I could do would stop it.

Daniel:	Have you seen those girls in the paper who have been playing footy?
GT:	Oh yeah, yeah …
Daniel:	Yeah, her brother … she plays cricket too.
Paul:	Yeah, I've seen two [fights]. I've seen the one between Johnno and Thompson.
Stephen:	See, this is where guys aren't very smart — they don't understand that beating the crap out of each other just because they can or to see who is better is completely pointless because then you're both in pain for the next few days.
Daniel:	Your war between a wog group and an Australian group would really be that hostile.
GT:	So there aren't many fights?
Paul:	There's usually a couple a year.
Daniel:	I don't know what happens when you get out of the school because we have a fairly iron principle about that.
Paul:	I spoke to Robert, he was in Werribee, and supposedly there was a fight every second day, and he's got this huge scar with four pin pricks because someone came at him with a fork.
Miread:	Our school isn't very rough … we're all real pussies. If our guys go on an excursion and there are all these other schools there, they'll say, 'Yeah, we'll start a fight' and then as soon as they fight back, they'll whimper.
Paul:	Yeah, it's all a big pose … these guys are just like, 'We'll start a fight' and then they're all whimpery …
Stephen:	Which brings back how stupid guys are — let's start a fight because we can.
Daniel:	As far as social groups go, I don't really have one … I sort of have friends in all of them … so I don't really get … that mentality. I don't have a wog or Australian mentality or any other kind.

It's clear from these comments that the 'wog' group has a definite presence at the school and is associated by these students with a particular type of behaviour rather than with a particular place of origin. There is an accent, there is smoking, and there is a projection of toughness. In Australia, the 'wog' is similar to the north American 'gino' and a form of 'in your face' otherness. Miread's comments that girls she has known for years make a conscious decision to speak in a particular way as part of adopting this identity. There is an association between being a 'wog' and being European. The only origin they name is Russian, and the boy in question is characterised by what is seen as an incongruent relationship between his height and tough persona. Wogs are seen as 'arrogant' and as having a 'separate hierarchy'. The stakes are high with even the 'most popular cheerleader' appearing like 'dirt' within the sovereign state of 'wogdom'. These students are not associated with academic competency. Here, their only engagement with the rest of the school community seems to be through the demarcation disputes over seats in the smoking zone in the far reaches of the school playing fields. Indeed, the main fights witnessed by these students have been between the wogs and the jocks. In this context, the jocks (and their sisters) are associated with cricket and Australian-rules football. They are 'big' and 'horrible'. Miread's comment that the 'wog chicks' have their 'wog guys' and treat Aussie girls with contempt makes obvious the heterosexual underpinning of these subcultures. In this context, it is 'Aussie' that is used derogatively. There is clear reference to the negative derivation of the term 'wog' and its current strident use in a form of identity politics that responds to exclusion through exclusion. Neither the wogs nor the jocks are held in high regard — this is not a politics of envy. Indeed, these groups are treated with even more contempt because in reality they are 'pussies' who 'whimper' in the company of boys from schools where kids are truly tough. Stephen links fighting to a particular form of masculinity that is pointless and stupid. Daniel and Paul attempt more sympathetic insights into the jocks, but by the end of this sequence distance themselves from it and confirm once again that they don't identify with a particular group and further to this, are happy to socialise with a range of students.

In-Between Spaces

GT: And are you lot typical? Like are there lots of other people like you here or are most people in a group?

Paul: There are a lot that choose a group but would easily talk to somebody else.

Daniel: It's not like Year 7 or Year 8, it was very ... everyone had a group.

Stephen: Which stuffed up when our group broke up.

GT: So what was your group in Year 7?

Stephen: I was in Daniel's group, and we had a massive group; it was like twenty people and then after Year 8, it split in half and those halves just crumbled ... it just fell.

Daniel: We had some that just went straight down into the depths of the geek world, and then you had ones that went off to be bigger better people ...

Miread: From younger years I was a part of the blonde group ... and I was perhaps more blonde ...

Daniel: We used to think she was evil.

Miread: Everyone stereotypes me because everyone thought I was bitchy. Oh, no ... none of them ever bothered to have a conversation with me, but they all knew that ...

Stephen: Because we were afraid of your friends! It's like, 'Oh, can't talk to them, they're too good for us'.

Miread: I feel for the girls that get stereotyped, because I got it really bad, and now I'm sort of friends with everybody, and people say, 'Oh, I used to hate you', and I'm like 'Oh, well … thanks, not that you knew me!' And they'd say. 'Oh, you just looked like a cow'. Yeah, so there's a lot of stereotyping with everyone … especially when you're younger.

Daniel: But then when you get to senior school, it changes so much. Like, I said before, the younger year levels have their stereotyping it sort of goes away a bit in senior school, and your teachers become more friends not evil people telling you what to do. And there's a huge difference between younger and older year levels.

GT: Do you have to go because I can talk for hours …

Stephen: I can stay a bit longer.

GT: Describe punk …

Daniel: These are musos.

Paul: These were people who were nice young people, majority were nice Jewish girls and now they've heard one punk music thing and are dressing up like …

Stephen: They're into heavy metal, rock, they wear chains …

Miread: They're fashionably angry. It's like, 'We hate the world, this is so bad …'.

Daniel: 'I'm unique, just like everybody else!'

Stephen: It's quite pathetic.

Daniel: Officially, that's my group … I suppose.

Miread: Nah.

Stephen: No, you're not … you're not a punk.

Daniel: But I spend all my time with them at recess … I don't know why but I did …

Paul: I'm going on language exchange and the majority of them are punks … they're real punks. They're not amazingly out there unless they're going to a punk concert, but they're real punks. The nonconformist type who listen to only punk music and rebel against everything. Then you have these wannabe, try-hard punks.

Stephen: The chicks at our school who wear the clothes …

Paul: Who are dressing over the top everyday — the black and the …

Daniel: Ilana was a nice Jewish girl; I went to her Bar Mitzvah and nowadays she wears a collar with studs on it. But she still walks around being a nice Jewish girl but with a collar.

Miread: Yeah, it's just a stage because I went through it.

Daniel: But you went through it before anyone else.

Miread: I had my little rebellious stage.

[two girls come into view]

Daniel: Oh, here's Amy.

Miread: Amy!

Stephen: And Nadine ... those are two you need to have in your group.

Miread: Do you want me to get them?

Daniel: Yeah, get them.

These four students enjoyed the interview and provided a range of insights that indicated their levels of maturity and sophistication relative to other interviewees. The flow of conversation was indicative of both their generosity and their intellectual energy. They did not consider themselves typical of groups of students at the school and indicated that I should interview others who were not like them. The two girls who entered the room at the end of this interview were targeted by Stephen as worthy of interviewing. Nadine and Amy came into the room because they wanted to know what was going on and stated that they did not want to be left out. I followed this up and it was not until after the interview with these two girls that the comment 'those are two you need' played out its full resonance. Stephen and the others knew that these girls would provide very different insights and had typecast them as 'blonde' girls. The flow of the interview in my experience makes almost as much of a statement as the words and the meanings attributed to them. Compared to these four students, Amy and Nadine's interview, was less free flowing. In the context of them initiating the interview, this came as a surprise. In some ways, the two girls were being set up by their own reluctance to be left out. This will be discussed further in the following chapter.

Daniel, Stephen, Paul, and Miread did not wholly commit to any one label. Stephen understood that he could be constructed as 'geek', which was linked to academic competency, in part through his participation in the accelerated learning program. He described his 'social status' in a way that assumed a low standing in the hierarchy. In his mind, this was linked to being a 'geek' and homosexual and juxtaposed most starkly to the 'jocks' and 'wogs', boys who represented particular forms of masculinity. His relationships with 'popular' girls in particular brought out his feelings of vulnerability at the hands of 'their guy friends'. Miread, Paul, and Daniel also used 'geek' to describe themselves, but qualified this as 'humanities geek' or 'band geek'. They weren't the traditional 'science geeks' and their capacity to socialise was used by implication to justify this positioning. Miread's defence of the 'blonde' girls, despite the others' clear fear and contempt for this group, provided vivid insights into the power this group had to make others 'feel like shit' and therefore intimidate them. It also provided insights into the fact that even within this seemingly powerful group, students felt vulnerable. Here was a politics of envy, which targeted and labelled these girls as 'bitchy' when in Miread's terms it was others who behaved in the way they were accused of behaving. She complained bitterly about the stereotypes based on ignorance, the fact that no one had bothered to talk to her and seemed not to engage directly with Stephen's comment that this was because he was afraid of her friends. At one stage, Daniel claims the 'label' punk, but is told in no uncertain terms that despite his socialising with the punks he cannot claim the label. Real punks are really angry, while 'wannabe' punks are fashionably angry. Clearly, Daniel is neither. Miread, on the other hand, has been blonde, punk, and humanities geek. Having completed her 'rebellious stage' she was now moving on.

These four students, despite their various social positionings, were close friends and had remained so over many years. They were a tremendous source of support for each other and bemoaned the fact that the school had split them up through timetabling. Stephen noted his isolation in English, for example, where he was without his friends and in a class with bullying jocks. Daniel created the image of 'pods' of junior school students and speaks to how this no longer exists in more senior years. These 'pods' are described variously as sources of community and support and as zones of unproductive demarcation. An illustration of the paradox of community. These students described subcultures that existed at the school and linked these to various levels of academic prowess. In their minds, some groups were clearly academically competent. Other groups were not. The wogs, for example, were represented as unquestionably low performing. They positioned the jocks and blondes as academically low performing and then discussed whether or not this stereotype was justified. The 'Asians' were represented as clearly academic. Miread, Stephen, Paul, and Daniel had their love of learning in common and also their reluctance to identify with any one group. The relationship between identity in these terms and academic achievement will be explored through interviews with 'wog chicks' and 'blonde' girls, groups identified by these four students as low academic achievers.

Chapter 7

Choosing to Perform — 'Wogs' and 'Blondes'

> The wogs are generally kind of gangster types, that's the way I see it. And I don't know too much about them, so I can't say too much. The thing that surprised me about them is that they don't have to be European. Most of the time you think of wogs as Greeks or Italians, but the group of wogs in my year level though mostly Greek and Italian like most wogs, it has a presence of other very different ethnicities, for example, Chinese, there's one guy I know from Iran, I think.
>
> (Dimitri, Year 9)

A major interest in my exploration of identification is the relationship between attributed identities, owned, identities and performed identity. The various emphasis given to attributed, owned, and performed identity is responsive to a range of factors including the particular school culture. In this regard, some students have more room to move than others. In the case of students who are deemed 'Asian' for example, because of a range of physical characteristics, identity choices are circumscribed in particular ways. The ability to choose identity is itself a marker of privilege. The relationship between how students appear to others and how they characterise their position within a school is both situated and fluid. A great deal seems to rest on performing what is understood to be 'popular' or 'wog' behaviour and in the case of some students this performance becomes more or less difficult. In the case of 'wogs', their decision to own the label has become a form of identity politics. Their parents, however, were called 'wogs' as a term of ridicule and abuse. However, for such young people there is also a cost in not identifying as 'wogs'. Some students who had a Greek background, for example, spoke of experiences of harassment when they refused to identify as 'wogs'. This was seen as an act of betrayal, a refusal to stand up and be counted as one of 'us' — an 'us' that was not popular. Other students described the 'wogs' as arrogant — an arrogance forged arguably through discourses of two-way exclusion. In a similar way, being a 'blonde' girl was tied up with performing a set of behaviours. Actual blondeness was not a prerequisite. However, the cost of entry into this popular group was being labelled 'bitchy' and 'ditzy', labels some students associated with the politics of envy. In ways such as these, the school subcultures were real and yet in other ways they stood in the students' imaginations. So, many students identified the subcultures and what characterised them and yet found it difficult to place themselves within them. Instead, naming real people as members of subcultures required closer scrutiny that illustrated how subcultures were stereotypes that were challenged by the individuals within them. Students came to combine characteristics associated with various subcultures and in this way placed themselves between rather than within them.

In Chapter 6, four students who were both academically successful and diverse in various ways were described. These students were reticent to own a label, but provided insightful descriptions of the subgroups that they perceived operated at their school. In broad terms, they identified themselves as 'nerds' of one type or another — 'humanities nerd' or 'band nerd' but in so doing stretched beyond recognition the original meaning they had given to 'nerd'. During the final stages of the interview, two girls came into the room demanding to know who I was and what was happening. The four students being interviewed suggested that these were girls I *had* to interview. This section draws on two separate interviews, one with these two girls, Amy and Nadine, who were described by other students as 'popular' or 'blonde' girls. The other interview was with Sophia, Anna, and Lucy who were characterised as 'wogs' by other students.

Relative to other interviews, these two were the least free flowing. The 'nerds' and the 'musos' understandings of the range of issues with which I am concerned was sophisticated and their immediate readiness to engage with these issues made for easy flowing and enjoyable interviews. Whilst not wishing to overinterpret the interview dynamic, it would be naive to ignore how some groups of students were able to make the interview their own. After a few prompts from me, these students were able to take the interview where they wanted it to go, while others were happy to provide short responses only, which in turn prompted me to ask a great many more questions. It is important to consider how students' behaviour during the interview speaks to the identity issue as well as to power. Relative noncompliance can be read as a form of resistance, even when the interview has been prompted by the interviewees. Perhaps 'nerds' and 'musos' are more adept at interacting with adults and honing in on their priorities and frames of reference. In other words, how do students from various subcultures perform the interview differently and how does my version of the good interview presume high levels of cultural capital?

As an interviewer I had to work harder to get responses from the five girls described here. This relative lack of easy dialogue was an outstanding aspect of the interview with Amy and Nadine, given they had been the initiators of the interaction. Sophia, Anna, and Lucy seemed to let things wash over them. Nadine and Amy created a very different impression. Amy and Nadine were forthright and were the only students to seek me out. Their ability to be 'plugged in' — to know what was going on at the school — was a critical aspect of their self-projection as was their capacity to make things happen. The interview process made this evident. Having approached me, I made it clear that they would need their teacher's permission to be absent from class and parental permission to be involved in the study. Within ten minutes they came back with a note from their coordinator stating they could attend the interview. They suggested I phone their parents for their permission and presented me with their mobile phones after dialling. They assured me that the signed consent form would be at the school the next day when I informed them that this verbal consent could only act as a temporary measure. They were true to their word. This process left me with the strong impression that these were girls in control. I had taken for granted that their instigation of the interview meant they were interested in talking with me. On reflection, I have come to understand that wanting to be interviewed is quite distinct from wanting to talk. They did not want to miss out on something that was going on. They wanted to be seen to be involved. Perhaps in their eyes, being interviewed had some status. It was difficult for me to resist the temptation to see Nadine as performing the disengaged schoolgirl. She seemed intent on camouflaging an element of who she was behind a veneer of feigned disinterest. In many ways the interview became part of the performance of being 'blonde'.

Interview transcripts are not flavoured by intonation, body language, and nonverbal communication between interviewees and between interviewees and the interviewer. In the case of Nadine and Amy, these issues were most pronounced. Amy and Nadine seemed to finish each other's sentences, but it was Amy who gave the impression of deferring to Nadine through eye contact and a 'wait and see' stance with regard to her comments. They were interviewed on the same day as Miread, Daniel, Stephen, and Paul. They were planning their

Year 11 subjects after interviews with the senior school coordinators. However, unlike the students discussed in Chapter 6, they made little mention of the school subcultures in direct ways.

GT:		Which students do well at school?
Amy:		Smart ones.
Nadine:		I don't want to be racist, but Asians do. They're just smart. Oh, I think they work hard as well. Also, the people that are naturally smart, they succeed.
Amy:		The people that do their work …
Nadine:		The people that aren't lazy succeed.
Amy:		Don't leave their homework till the last minute.
Nadine:		People who prioritise their education over their social life.
GT:		Are you in that category?
Nadine:		No!
Amy:		We try …
Nadine:		Around exams we are … but if it's not near exams and there's a choice of doing homework or going out, I'll go out. I don't stay home to study when I can do something else.
GT:		What do you do when you go out … I mean what's going out?
Nadine:		Parties … yeah.
Amy:		Walking around … not much.
GT:		And you're in Year 11 next year, are you looking forward to that?
Nadine:		Not really, no!
GT:		Why?
Amy:		Too much work.
Nadine:		We had our interviews and they said, 'You're going to have heaps of work with the subjects you've chosen for next year'.
Amy:		Yeah.

Nadine and Amy are straightforward about the students who they think do well at school. High achievers are naturally smart, work hard, and prioritise their schoolwork over their social life. In the case of the 'Asians' these categories are conflated in their eyes. There exists a discourse whereby naming 'Asian' students as successful is deemed dangerous and the statement by Nadine that she doesn't want to appear racist reflects this discourse. It is worth considering why naming the category 'Asian' and linking it to success can be deemed racist. Is the very naming of this racialised group dangerous? Or perhaps it is linking it with academic success, which is dangerous, given the implication that being academic excludes the possibility of being 'popular'? More likely these students have internalised a way of understanding 'Asian' students that positions them as successful and therefore threatening to other students. This is what Hage (1998) refers to as Asians as 'superhuman' and by implication, a way of furthering the 'us and them' divide and moreover, consolidating the 'them' as dangerous. When asked if they are successful students, Nadine and Amy equivocate. The immediate response to this question is an emphatic 'no' — social life comes before school life. However, on closer examination, their negative response is qualified. They describe how school work takes priority before exams, as it does when there is nothing better to do. Through the words of their teachers, they describe the Year 11 subjects they have chosen as those that require a lot of work. Later in the interview when they were asked directly about their marks, their response confirms that academic achievement is a priority. They were achieving A's and B+'s, which they described as average.

GT: B+ and A isn't average!

Nadine: Yeah, but ... like ... this year and last semester I just sort of missed out on the mark above ... I probably could get better if I tried, but ...

Amy: I don't think I did very well on my exams ...

Nadine: Yeah, you can always say that you can do better. But we just happened to have a lot better to do!

Nadine's statement that they 'have a lot better to do' implied both that they had better things to do than school work and lots of room for improving their school work. It was an apt way of summing up what I took to be an ambivalent representation of themselves as social not academic. Nadine, in particular, seemed to be pacing herself. She knew she had more to give academically and had a canny sense of when it was most important to do so.

There appears little substance to their out-of-school social life, which is constituted as 'parties', 'walking around' and 'not much'. Social life at school, by comparison, is described in more detail. Nadine and Amy go into detail about how hierarchies of friends are constituted through what might appear to others as the relatively trivial nuances of who initiates corridor contact.

GT: So you don't put yourselves into groups?

Nadine: Yeah, well we have a group of friends, but I wouldn't say it was like a definite group, like …

Amy: Because there's a lot of people who have a couple of their friends in one group but are still good friends with others … I don't know it's weird.

Nadine: Yeah, well you've got your best friends and they don't really change much and then there's sort of like your good friends who sort of … you don't really arrange to see them. Like, if you're going out with your best friends then they won't be there, but something bigger, you'll see them and then there's just the people who are your friends but you …

Amy: Yeah, you wouldn't go and make an effort to say 'Hi' in the corridor.

Nadine: Yeah, you wouldn't go out with them.

GT: And what about at school? Do you hang around with a group of kids at lunchtime?

Nadine: It's kind of changed … the canteen's gone!

Amy: When the canteen was there, everyone used to just go there and hang out, and everyone just stands in a group and talks to everyone, and now we have nowhere to go!

Nadine: It used to be everyone around the canteen pretty much.

Amy: Because all the year levels go there.

Nadine: And you just mingle with everyone, and now that it's gone we're sort of lost. We had nowhere to go, so we just resorted to out the front with just the girls.

Amy: And the guys didn't …

Nadine: Yeah, the guys were really immature, so we don't really hang around them much … but yeah, the last few weeks we felt lost!

GT: So when you go out on the weekend, are there guys in your group or do you …

Amy: There's like a couple that we've been friends with since Year 7 and who we go out with at a party or something.

GT: But the guys that you just called immature are at the parties too?

Amy: They're our good friends but they're immature!

Nadine: Yeah. And every now and then we'll go out with other guys that aren't them, because they just piss us off because they're so immature!

Amy: And they get angry that we go out with other guys.

Nadine: But they're allowed to hang out with younger girls … and they get angry at us if we're friends with other guys.

Amy:	They're all friends with the Year 9 girls.
Nadine:	Because ... just because they're all sluts ... and they get angry at us. Like last year, when we were really good friends with all the grammar school guys and we saw them heaps and they got really pissed off at us for doing that, so then they became friends with the Year 9s!
GT:	Oh ok, so I see, the Year 10 boys hang around with the Year 9 girls and the Year 10 girls hang around with the Year 10 boys ...
Nadine:	From other schools, and then this year we sort of got friends with the Year 11s and 12s ...
Amy:	Because the Year 12s have brothers in our year level as well ...

This exchange provides interesting insights into heterosexual dynamics between year levels. The boys in their year level (Year 10) are immature but good friends. Yet Nadine and Amy are concerned that these same boys get angry with them when they interact with boys at more senior year levels. This interaction takes place almost as 'revenge' given the Year 10 boys' interactions with Year 9 'sluts'. In a few short statements, these girls evoke a sexual double standard that implies a set of unequal and gendered power relations. Their response is to denigrate the younger girls rather than act on the boys' behaviour described as 'immature' and 'angry'. It is worth reviewing Stephen's descriptions of the same dynamics; in this context. Stephen, discussed in Chapter 6, stressed the power 'popular' kids, including the girls, had to make others 'feel like shit', these girls seemed less aware of their use of power. They competed with younger girls for the boys' attention and seemed to be playing off groups of boys against each other. The Year 10 boys at their own school were the ones of least interest to them; immature and interested in the Year 9 girls, the senior boys at their school were more attractive as were the boys from the nearby elite grammar school before they became friends with the Year 9 'sluts'. Yet what is also clear through this exchange is the pivotal place boys occupy in the way girls define their own and each other's social status.

GT:	So you're generally happy at school?
Nadine:	Yeah ... I really didn't want to come here in Grade 6; I really wanted to go to a private school ... but
Amy:	My mum was going to send me to the nearby Catholic girls' school and I really didn't want to go ... it's like a Catholic school ...
Nadine:	Yeah, I really didn't want to come here you know — 'I don't want to go to a public school'.
Amy:	I didn't know that!

Nadine:	Now I look back and basically — apart from ... the only thing I think it lacks is that private schools have weekend sports and they have a lot more activities, that's another thing I'd change ... putting that in the curriculum or something, but otherwise, basically it has high standards and everything and it's a pretty good school, so yeah.
Amy:	I reckon I could do better here than if I went to a girls' school.
GT:	Is that the reason you came here instead of the Catholic girls' school?
Amy:	It was probably one of the reasons ... because all the girls there get distracted by that because they're not at school with them [boys] and so they aren't used to being around them.
Nadine	Yeah, it's good because everyone here ... there's no people who are really up themselves and it's probably got a lot to do with their economic status ... there's no one here that's extremely rich or spoilt.

Here, the two girls speak to separate agendas. For Amy, private schools are symbolised by the local Catholic girls school that attracts modest fees. Being Catholic and being single sex is what she dislikes. She reiterates the discourse that girls at single-sex schools overreact to boys because they are not used to them. The other side of the coin is the statement that girls at coeducational schools are distracted by boys and underachieve. Either way, girls are positioned as reactive and the assumed central place of boys in their lives is reiterated. Nadine, on the other hand, focuses on elite private and coeducational schools noted for their weekend activities. She states that Leafy Suburbs College is better because of the lack of the 'extremely rich or spoilt'. She is the only student to mention socioeconomic issues in a direct way. Academic standards remain her priority and given these are high at Leafy Suburbs College, she is happy with the school. It is guesswork as to whether Nadine would have been happier at a private school and whether this was a real choice for her family. If so, her preferences had been well camouflaged, up until this point, given Amy's surprise at Nadine's statement that she had not wanted to attend a public school.

A relative lack of free-flowing discussion was also a feature of the interview with the other group of girls. Anna, Katrina, and Lucy were interviewed together on a separate occasion. In their case, I came to understand their fewer words as symptomatic of their having little to say in general. These girls complained about school being too hard, of teachers expecting too much, and in a similar way perhaps, I as the interviewer was expecting them to do more than they were willing. Anna, Katrina, and Lucy were in the beginning stages of Year 10 at the time of the interview. It was Lucy's last day at the school. She was moving to Alternative Collage, a nearby government school. She had come to Leafy Suburbs College from another school, making it her third secondary college in almost as many years. Her first school was the neighbourhood Catholic girls' college mentioned by Amy. Anna, Sophia, and Lucy did not give the impression that their relationship to each other was as close as that of Nadine and Amy. Nor did any one girl seem to be in charge in the same way as Nadine seemed. They were comfortable with each other and stated that they were closely involved as friends in and out of school.

Amy, Nadine, and Lucy presented as mainstream Australian, Sophia was of Greek background and Anna identified her mother as Maltese and made no mention of her father. Anna, Sophia, and Lucy had been described to me as 'wogs'. Just as 'blondes' did not have to be blonde, 'wogs' did not have to have a history of migration. Some 'real' Australians chose to hang around with 'wogs' and Lucy was in this category. Had other students not nominated these girls as 'wogs' I would not have recognised them as such. It is noteworthy that the term 'wog' is most often centred on boys and constructed around their particular interpretation of masculinity (Martino and Pallotta-Chiarolli 2001, 2003). One teacher commented 'girls don't really identify themselves as wogs.' Within Australia the 'wog' image has come to the fore through popular culture, particularly television comedy, often performed by the children of postwar immigrants and referred to as 'ethnic humour'. Particular characters have been popularised and the 'wog' girl is personified through the character of Effie. Effie had appeared in various plays and TV shows. At the time of the study, she was appearing in a commercial for a telephone company and headed a television show entitled 'Greeks on the Roof', which was based on the British show *The Kumars at No. 11* featuring an Indian family. In the show, Effie in the company of her parents and brother, interviews various celebrities. Effie is portrayed by an actor of Greek origin. Effie is the daughter of Greek immigrants. She is loud, self-assured, chews gum, and speaks a form of ungrammatical English that has both working-class and Greek-Australian undertones. Her dress and hair are flamboyant in a way that denotes an unsophisticated 'look at me' style. The alternative image of the 'wog' girl is that of timidity. The 'good' Greek girl is overprotected and policed in relation to a family politics of honour (Tsolidis 1995 2003; Bottomley 1979, 1992). These images of Greek women coincide with the characters in *My Big Fat Greek Wedding*, which was also popular at the time of the study. This film portrays the life of a North American woman of Greek origins and her attempts to integrate her 'Greek' self into a new way of being. This revolves around her relationship with a man who does not have a Greek background. This film rehearses many of the issues central to depictions of ethnic minorities in countries such as America, Australia, and Canada. These include the nature of the family and within it the role of women (Tsolidis 2001). The 'wog' girl is either like the overprotected main character of the film, who is struggling to find a space outside her family, or she is like the overprojected bride's cousin, who is very self-assured. In the context of such representations of the 'wog' girl, it may not be surprising that 'girls don't readily identify themselves as wogs'. Sophia, Anna and Lucy did not sound or look like Effie. The interview began with discussion of Lucy's imminent departure from Leafy Suburbs College. She explained that she wanted to change schools in the following way:

Lucy:	Um … because I want to do Hospitality and you can't do it here so I had to move to a school that does do it. So, yeah.
GT:	And are you looking forward to that?
Lucy:	Um, yeah, a bit.
GT:	What aren't you looking forward to?
Lucy:	Leaving friends here and making a new start again.

Lucy had begun her secondary schooling at a Catholic girls' school. Whilst this girls' school is a private school, only modest fees are required. It is highly sought after, having developed a strong reputation for being supportive and encouraging of girls. Lucy did not provide any insights into why she had left the Catholic school. She did state that it had been less demanding of her than Leafy Suburbs College. The move from Leafy Suburbs College was prompted by a curriculum choice that dovetailed with a vocational interest. Hospitality was not part of the strictly academic repertoire of subjects offered at Leafy Suburbs College. Nothing Lucy said implied that the move was responsive to teacher counselling. Lucy's statement that Leafy Suburbs College was strict and demanded academic rigour were echoed by the other girls.

Sophia began these girls' responses to my question about groupings of students at the school.

Sophia:	Everyone talks to each other, and you've got like enemies and stuff, but there are heaps of different groups.
GT:	Do you recognise those groups by a name?
Anna:	There's like the 'smokers' and, like, and the 'hardcores' and they go down the back [oval] and they don't really care about anyone else. And they'll bag people and start fights and stuff, and then there's another group which is like the main group and they're friendly nice and everyone's … most of us are a big group and have parties together and things like that. And then there's …
Sophia:	That Russian group …
Lucy:	Yeah, the Russians. They're just girls and they stick together …
GT:	And they're all Russian?

Lucy:	Yeah.
GT:	And are they new to the country?
Anna:	No …
Sophia:	They've been here since Year 7, they're just Russian!
Lucy:	They're a bit up themselves and snobby and think they're better than everyone else.
GT:	Oh, ok. And do they speak in Russian?
Sophia:	Yeah.
Lucy:	Sometimes, just between them.
Sophia:	There's a group of boys who … the big group, the boys who always play four-square. The boys aren't really friends with each other, but they all come together and play four-square.
Lucy:	It's nice that they're like that.
GT:	And how do these groups do academically? Are they good at school or bad at school?
Anna:	Not necessarily …
Sophia:	It depends.
Anna:	I think they all vary. I'd say most of the Russian girls I'd say are smart,
Sophia	But they're smart in some things.
Lucy:	Because a lot of them do Year 11 subjects now, and a few of them that don't.
Anna:	And the people that go down the back oval, some are smart, and some are really failing. Everyone's just different. I don't really know, it just depends who you have classes with I guess. You don't know what everyone's like.
GT:	What I'm hearing is that there are subgroups, like social groups, but that doesn't necessarily tell you if they're good at school … is that right?
Anna:	Yeah.
GT:	So what kids are good at school?
Sophia:	I think lots of Asian kids are. Maybe not so in English, but maths and all other subjects. A lot of them are sent out from their country and stay with their guardian, and they study here, there are a few in our class.
GT:	Where do they come from?
Sophia:	I think one's from … Hong Kong. She's sent out to finish school here. She's in Year 10 and she's doing Year 12 maths. She's really smart. All she seems to do is study heaps.

GT:	What other sort of kids are good at school? Are there other kids that stand out as good students?
Anna:	Yeah, there's people that stand out because they're smart or whatever and they get awards or achievements. I don't think it's necessarily a type though, I think it just depends on how determined and focused you are and how smart you are, I don't know.
GT:	And does it work the same way the other end — is there a type that isn't good.
Lucy:	I think it just depends, you could think that they're not smart, but then you find out that they're actually smarter than you make them out to be. So it all just depends on what you see kind of thing.
GT:	And does it work that way for girls and boys or is it different?
Anna:	It's the same.

As with other students, these girls identify most expansively as distinct groups within the school, those most commonly ethnicised; the Russians, because they speak another language and 'stick together', and the 'Asian' students. Both these groups are understood to be high academic achievers. Here there is reference to students who live with their guardians, a comment that presumably refers to international students. Lucy, Sophia, and Anna are unclear as to the reasons why some students achieve — there is reference to studying at the expense of other activities, natural ability, and determination and focus. There is also the astute observation that there can be a difference between how a student appears out of class relative to what type of student they are in class. According to Lucy, 'It all just depends on what you see', which is profound in a seemingly simple way. These girls also mention the 'hardcores', the smokers who start fights at the back of the oval. However, unlike other students, they do not identify 'wogs' in this context. They also mention the boys who play four-square as a group worth noting. These are boys constituted at the other end of the spectrum relative to the 'popular' boys. This game is a noncontact game where players hit a ball using their hands into squares painted onto the ground. It does not sit comfortably with dominant images of masculinity as these are tied to football, cricket, or soccer.

GT:	And what do you kids do out of school?
Anna:	Go out, parties ... work.
GT:	What do you do work-wise?
Anna:	I work in a retail store in [local shopping centre]. I work most weekends, Saturday and Sunday during the day, and I usually go out on a Saturday night with friends.

GT:	Anyone do sport or anything like that?
Sophia:	Yeah, tennis on Saturday mornings and I train on Wednesday night for half an hour.
GT:	How about you?
Lucy:	I play basketball; yeah, that takes up Sunday night.
GT:	So what sorts of bands or TV shows do you like watching?
Anna:	I like most TV shows, *Big Brother*, all those *Australian Idol* and all those reality ones … and the soapies, the *OC* …

These girls did not place themselves into any particular student subculture. They described their social lives as revolving around parties. Sophia was involved with tennis and Lucy with a basketball team. In addition, Anna mentioned working in retail on Saturdays and Sundays. This was presented with little weighting, almost as an afterthought. Yet the time commitment of working two full days a week must have been significant. Anna's comment brought to the fore the real socioeconomic differences between students. Whether she worked by choice or necessity was left in abeyance, but her comment was the only one of its kind, bringing to life the very real issue of how some students are in situations where they do need to contribute to their and their family's economic survival. This needs to be considered in relation to academic achievement. One teacher noted that students who succeed academically

> have to have that independence, you know, to choose to want to work, but you have to be focused. If they're focused, they'll pass — if they're not focused, they won't. If they spend too much time doing other things like part-time work or you know with a boyfriend or girlfriend, they're not going to pass.

Sophia had mentioned her Greek background early in the interview. Later in the interview, I raised this issue again.

GT:	And do you think being Greek has made a difference? Or your parents being Greek? Do you see yourself as Greek?
Sophia:	Sort of, I was born here, and I've been brought up with some cultural things, but I only do those when I'm told to. I won't go out of my way to do them.
GT:	What sort of things?
Sophia:	Like, Easter, name days and stuff like that … if my mum tells me. Even my parents don't really …
Anna:	Will you do it when you get older?
Sophia:	Probably …

Anna:	(laughs)
Sophia:	... to my kids ... but like ... because my parents have been brought up by people off the boat.
GT:	But your parents were born here?
Sophia:	Oh, my dad wasn't — he was born overseas, but he moved here when he was five. But, yeah, I'll probably do the same thing.
GT:	And do you speak Greek?
Sophia:	Yeah, and Greek school and stuff.
GT:	You go now? So will you be doing Greek as a Year 11 or Year 12 subject?
Sophia:	Um ... nah, it's really difficult. The grammar and the tenses are like French, they're really complicated.
GT:	So are you doing a language here?
Sophia:	Nope ...
Anna:	Nah ...
Lucy:	No.
GT:	And were your parents born here?
Anna:	Yeah. My mum's Maltese ...
GT:	So does that flow into your life at all?
Anna:	Not really.

Sophia described a range of activities commonly associated with Greekness. She attended a community-based Greek school out of school hours, spoke the language, and adhered to some traditions. Despite her protestations that this was done only under duress, she confirmed that these were all aspects of her life she would continue into the future and with her own children. This is not uncommon, particularly within the Greek community, which has a strong history of diasporic cultural maintenance (Tsolidis 1995). Anna, by contrast, remained relatively untouched by her mother's cultural heritage, and her question to Sophia about her adherence to Greek cultural tradition seemed somewhat pointed in the context. Sophia was keen to distinguish herself from those 'off the boat'. This is a common means of indicating relative levels of Australian acculturation.

Anna, Sophia, and Lucy left me with an overwhelming impression of disengagement from the school culture. These were not the girls who were in the music and theatre program, the accelerated learning program, or particularly active in sport. Instead, they described their interests as fashion and Anna stated that, apart from working, her out-of-school interests centred on television, particularly reality shows and soapies. Explaining these girls' lives and ambitions through the cliché of 'waiting for Prince Charming' could be tempting. Instead, it may be worth contemplating how Lucy's decision to move to a school with a more vocational orientation would situate her relative to Sophia and Anna who were planning to remain at Leafy Suburbs College and do subjects that they understood as less demanding.

In the terminology used by these students, Stephen, Paul, Miread, and Daniel would be classified as 'nerds' or 'geeks' of one type or another. Anna, Sophia and Lucy were considered 'wog' girls and Nadine and Amy 'popular' or 'blonde' girls. Nonetheless, these three groups of students have a range of understandings in common. All note the Russian students as a visible group within the school. Despite being seen as 'wogs' by other students, Anna, Sophia, and Lucy show little empathy with the Russian girls. While Stephen, Paul, Miread, and Daniel understand their use of Russian in the context of their relative recency of arrival, these girls argue, instead, that having been in Australia since Year 7 provides little explanation for behaviour they read as exclusive and 'snobby'. It is also worth noting that Anna, Sophia, and Lucy identify the Russian group as consisting only of girls. Relative to Amy and Nadine and the others, the 'wog' girls seem most hostile toward the Russian girls, accusing them of arrogance and exclusivity. In a similar manner, Nadine and Amy's strongest comments are reserved for the Year 9 girls whom they describe as 'sluts'. It may be worth considering this in relation to rivalry between girls at a broader level. Miread speaks of 'bitchiness' as part of the stereotype of 'blonde' girls, but nonetheless confirms this form of interaction amongst other girls, who she argues are less secure about themselves. Bullying behaviour amongst girls is increasingly visible and has led some commentators to regard this as one of the disadvantages of single-sex schooling for girls (Bennett 2003). Ethnicity plays an important part in rivalry between girls and is illustrated by some of the comments made by students in this study. At Leafy Suburbs College the hierarchy of social groups was underpinned by heterosexual relations that positioned girls as subordinate to boys within each subculture. Yet the rivalry between these groups pitted particular girls against each other and particular groups of boys against each other. I have argued elsewhere that this is likely to make the most vulnerable group of girls more isolated and that this vulnerability and isolation can be linked to migrant status (Tsolidis 1986, 2001).

All three groups of interviewees I have described in Chapters 6 and 7 identified the 'Asian' students as a distinct group within the school. They were said to be academically competent, particularly in maths. The students interviewed, linked Asian students' academic prowess to parental pressure, including for those students who were in Australia without their parents. Sometimes this pressure is linked to a form of lacking. The children of immigrant parents are often seen as shouldering the burden of their own aspirations, those of their parents, as well as the responsibility of making worthwhile the dislocation and struggle that is often part of the migration experience (Tsolidis 2001). At Leafy Suburbs College, elements of this narrative are retold by students who appear to have very little real engagement with these 'Asian' students. Again the students with some familial, if not direct, experience of migration do not differentiate themselves from the other students in this regard. It is clear that the 'Russians' and the 'Asians' are Othered, including by students whose own background includes a history of migration.

Listening to Anna and Sophia describe their own lives and imagined futures as well as their understandings of the Russian girls hinted at the possible advantage of being an immigrant relative to the child of an immigrant. Anna and Sophia described the Russian girls as 'smart' and focused on successfully completing their schooling, comments that implied the impetus for upward social mobility and what has been described controversially as an alternative work ethic for migrant groups (Birrell and Seitz 1986). This seems a world away from Anna and Sophia and students like them, for whom participation in higher education is less likely than it was for their parents.

Of the nine students described so far, only three were boys. 'Jocks' and 'wog' boys were persistently difficult to interview. The reasons why this may be the case needs to be considered. The girls were less well represented in the 'nerd' category within these interviews, yet the VCE results for the school indicate that girls do better than boys. In 2003, for example, of the students who received a score above 90, the number of girls was twice that of the boys. The school was struggling to keep the number of boys and girls level, with the number of boys close to 55% of the total population. Leafy Suburbs College encouraged a wide range of masculinities as acceptable within formal and informal activities. Boys performed in the school musical, in the choir, and orchestra. Girls and boys played the full range of instruments, perhaps with the exception of junior boys who seemed to dominate the specialist percussion ensemble. The emphasis on sport also allowed for a range of interests and the encouragement given to football and cricket was matched with enthusiasm for nontraditional sports such as cycling. Yet the girls' comments implied a set of traditional heterosexual underpinnings to interactions. The interview with Sophia, Anna, and Lucy finished with this exchange:

GT: The boys here are ok or do they give you a hard time?

Sophia: Some of them are ok; some of them think they're like king and crack smart-arse comments.

GT: So do they make you feel uncomfortable some of the boys?

Sophia: Probably more in Year 7 and 8, they used to, but now they're ok …

Anna: Yeah, we used to have problems … not problems just like … idiots being rude. I think everyone's sort of over it now. I think everyone's just friends now, no matter who you hang around with or whatever — you either like someone or hate them.

It is unreasonable to expect a school to eradicate attitudes and behaviours that are endemic in society more broadly. However, this short exchange reminds us that regardless of girls' academic success, there is still need to consider how we can provide all girls with a school space that is comfortable and safe. In a similar way, Stephen's comments, discussed in Chapter 6, highlight how traditional forms of masculinity and the femininities that respond to them also leave particular groups of boys vulnerable.

While subcultures were significant in framing students' understandings of identity, including with reference to academic achievement, it became increasingly evident that owning such identities was something keenly avoided by the students interviewed. As described in Chapter 6, Stephen explained that characterisations that created binaries between 'nerds' and 'cheerleaders' were 'an American television thing that they, used in the nineties to degrade people'. Perhaps instead, for these young people, 'Identities are for wearing and showing, not for storing and keeping' (Bauman 2004:89). In the next chapters several students who were identified as 'musos' will be described.

Chapter 8

'… Music Doesn't Really Cut It' — When Music Is and Isn't Your Life

A warm Saturday afternoon and the local street has been cordoned off with bright yellow plastic barriers. No car access means that the normally busy street, lined with small shops, is now filled with pedestrians. A makeshift stage has been set up at the far end of the area. A throng of people is visible at the side of the stage, mostly young people from the school. They wear white shirts and black skirts or trousers. Excitedly, they embrace each other and giggle with recognition as other individuals join the group. Their enthusiasm, energy, and enjoyment seem contagious. The small bus arrives and empties additional musicians onto the footpath. Students mix with the jumble of wires, instruments, and microphones and emerge on stage as the senior school band readies to perform at the local street festival. The boys have put on tailored jackets and in so doing have transformed themselves from schoolboys into young men. The girls wear the same jackets, but somehow these have less impact on their personas. The keyboard stands in front of Jake, an imposing young man whose blonde good looks, confidence, charisma, and extraordinary musical talent focuses attention. He holds the performance together with just the right combination of leadership and generosity of spirit toward the younger performers. At various intervals, the saxophonist, pianist and drummer perform solo, and as they do, the crowd of students listening clap and call their name. The enigmatic music teacher stands on the sidelines, clearly critical of the proceedings but peripheral to the performance. This is a 'feel good' occasion. These young people's talent and enthusiasm send a communal wave of admiration surging through the crowd of onlookers — a sort of confidence that our community will be safe in the hands of this generation.

For any researcher, Jake would be a 'must have' interviewee. He figured prominently in many school activities related to music and sport. He was in positions of leadership within the school. He was good looking and popular with students from many year levels. But coupled with this, he had a manner that was polite and open. He did not present as arrogant, but instead as someone who put others at ease. Amongst adolescent boys, it seemed a disarming combination of traits. Jake's father was the son of Greek immigrants; his mother was mainstream Australian. I assumed he would be both 'popular' and 'muso'. He was forthcoming in his readiness to be interviewed. This occurred in the final stages of Year 11 when he was in the process of finalising his selection of Year 12 subjects. He was also thinking about future careers, the qualifications he would need and subjects that were prerequisites for relevant courses. He made no mention of music and instead nominated either carpentry or natural medicine as his career choice. I asked about the absence of music.

> Yeah, I love it ... but I'm not going to do it because ... I'm still going to play gigs for sure and still practice ... but it's not the right sort of ... if I had my own way I'd do music but to do the things I love doing like surfing and windsurfing and water-skiing and skiing down slopes and stuff, I need that sort of money, and ... music doesn't really cut it ... but I'm still going to play gigs and stuff for sure, music's one of the biggest parts of my life definitely. (Jake)

For Jake, music was one of the biggest parts of his life and this was evident in the way he performed — both skill and passion. Anyone would have identified him first and foremost as a 'muso' and he was well aware of this being the way he was viewed. Yet in terms of his imagined future, it was his interest in sport that set the agenda. He needed money in order to pursue his sporting interests and therefore needed a job that could supply him with a stable and predictable source of income. Jake felt that he could not earn such an income through music. Money was a priority because sport was a priority and Jake nominated career paths distinct from sport and music as a means of earning an income. Jake was giving priority to sport over music and eliminating the possibility that either could provide him with satisfactory remuneration. This pessimism about music was evident in the comments of other students who identified as musos. This will be further discussed in subsequent chapters where students' imagined futures are further explored. In this chapter, I would like to provide insights into two interviews, one with Jake and the other conducted with two boys who were also in Year 11 at the time of the interview and identified as musos.

Jake was very positive about the school and the students. In contrast to the Year 10 students discussed in previous chapters, he expressed gratitude toward his teachers. Jake was aware of the hierarchy of subcultures and the intrigues that operated within and between these. Nonetheless, he felt that the hierarchies had minimal negative impact on students. Jake saw some of the same things others described, however, the significance he attached to them was quite different. I began the interview by asking Jake what sort of kids came to the school.

Jake:	I guess you've got like, the people who hang out and smoke and stuff, so you've got that kind of group. And you've got your sporty kids who are down on the back oval playing footy or whatever. You've got your musos who just hang out, and you've got a lot of different groups here.
GT:	And they get along with each other?
Jake:	Yeah, most of the time. I mean, you get little mingles all the time, but I guess it's part of school. But apart from that yeah, everyone's pretty chilled here.
GT:	What type of students do you think succeed at this school?
Jake:	Um, I don't reckon that if they smoke or if they hang out down the back and play sport all lunchtime, or if they play music it really hasn't got too much on if they succeed. I think it's more the kid's attitude. If the kid wants to like, you could have an absolute … a guy that smokes twenty packs a day or whatever and, he smokes pot as well or whatever and if he wants to do well at school, he will … or she. So I think it comes down to the attitude of the person, not so much yeah, what kind of kid it is.
GT:	So you think there isn't a group of kids at this school that do really, really well?
Jake:	Well, there's always the nerdy group, or the so-called nerdy group who are going to do really well.
GT:	Describe the nerdy group … what's the nerdy group?
Jake:	I guess …. it's a bit judgmental! But the people who, like you hear people don't have TVs they just get home they study, they have dinner they study, they get up in the morning and they study. I'd call that sort of …
GT:	Nerdy?
Jake:	Oh, you don't go round calling them … 'Oh yeah, you're a nerdy kid, go away' you just talk to them all, and you're mates with them all, but as far as it goes, they're sort of classified as the nerds.
GT:	And does it pay off? Like are they the ones that do really well?

Jake:	Um, I guess it would. They will do really well, because they put the time in. But yeah, I guess it comes down to time.
GT:	But they're not the only ones that do really well?
Jake:	No, no ...

Jake draws on the stereotype of 'nerds' as those who fill their lives with study at the expense of everything else, including TV. They put in the time and this pays off, but non-'nerds' can also do well at school. Jake describes himself as someone who should put more effort into his study, particularly English, which is not his strength.

> ... like, myself I'm not good at English but I'm really good at all the others, so I'll do a lot better in those than English. So it depends what area you're in ... I should do more work in English definitely! (Jake).

Jake links groups of students to groups of subjects in what would be seen as the traditional divide — 'nerds' and the sciences, 'cool' kids, and the arts. However, he qualifies his comment with the acknowledgment that this in itself may be a generalisation.

Jake:	They [nerds] tend to do the more sciency maths subjects, like Chem, Psych, um Physics all that kind of stuff. And I guess the people who aren't so nerdy, or the cool group — whatever you want to call them — will tend to do sort of, the art subjects. But that's a bit general as well because people might be really good at art who are nerdy or whatever so ...
GT:	So the music group doesn't do the same sort of subjects as each other?
Jake:	Nah, well, I do sport, I do PE, Bio, um ... Music, English, and Maths. Another girl — our bass player, she does um, she's an awesome artist and she does Visual Communication and Design, she did Studio Arts, she does Maths, she does Psych, so that sort of a ... yeah.

Jake remained ambivalent about what made a student academically successful. He was torn between the relative mix of what he described as 'raw talent' or 'genetics', and effort.

> Yeah, I reckon everyone's capable of doing it. Well, everyone's capable of doing their best, which might not be an A+. I guess it does come down to the genetics a bit, but I really still think if you put in the yards you'll get the result. (Jake)

In these comments, I could hear Jake struggling to reconcile the dominant school discourses linking achievement to effort and his lived experience of simply not being good at something, like English.

Asked what characterised the school, Jake responded in relation to his areas of interest.

Jake:	I guess it'd be the music and the sport. More so the sport these days, but it used to be the music, the music used to be awesome. We had some really talented players ... nowadays its still really good, but it's not as good as it used to be.
GT:	Why's that?
Jake:	I'm not, really not sure. There's a lot of talented players coming up now, but at the top end of the school there's not really a diverse big group of great players. Like, a couple of years ago there was a heap of great players, and it was just sort of like, 'Whoa, where do we go from here?' But, yeah that happens.
GT:	And the sport?
Jake:	The sport, I think, yeah ... I think that's growing.
GT:	Particular sports or generally?
Jake:	Um, I think generally. I think everyone's getting a bit more sporty these days I think. But I think it's a lot of things. I think they care what they look like, or social or ... pressure from parents, whatever it is, people are playing a lot more sport.
GT:	And is there a particular sport that happens ...?
Jake:	I guess, the footy, the basketball ... but also like rugby and netball and tennis ... so it's very diverse.
GT:	And kids like yourself are involved in both or is it divided?
Jake:	Not really ... Mr Ryan [music teacher] said to me at the swimming sports, 'Jake, you're not a real muso — musos can't play sport!' Yeah, so not many musos do play sport and vise versa.
GT:	Why do you think that's the case?
Jake:	I'm really not sure. Um ... yeah, not sure.
GT:	And is it the same for girls and boys?
Jake:	Nah, everyone's just together.
GT:	But there are girls represented in each?
Jake:	Oh yeah, definitely. And there's like girls footy and stuff ... and boys netball, so it's all mixed up and stuff.
GT:	All right ... so that's influenced your experience here, do you think? That's one of the things that's made it positive?

Jake: Yeah, definitely. Because I guess anytime you can get away from doing a bit of schoolwork and playing a bit of sport or music is always good. But yeah, it's really good. It sort of creates the school a lot more than studying. It can get kind of boring.

Leafy Suburbs College provided a wide range of activities for students, more than most government schools. For Jake, this was a clearly an aspect of the school that was important. He was not a standout academic performer and in his terms, music and sport provided interests that made school less 'boring'. Students can use 'boring' to describe something with which they have limited success. In the case of Jake, schoolwork is boring relative to sport and music.

Like other interviewees, Jake was reluctant to put himself into a particular school subculture. However, he conceded that

Jake: Other people would probably put me as a muso ...

GT: Yeah, but why would they do that?

Jake: Um ... because I spend a lot of time playing music. I'm in there, probably, four lunchtimes a week ... just sitting at the piano and just playing basically, so I guess the people that know me wouldn't really put me ... mates like Trevor and Johnno and that wouldn't put me in a group because I go mountain riding and play music and sort of ... but generally — people see me on stage — 'Oh yeah, he's a muso.'

GT: And what does a muso mean? Someone who spends a lot of time playing, or is it more than that?

Jake: Um, I don't know. See, for me, music's not just ... playing. It's sort of feeling. And I guess people can see that through my playing. Because I get in there and I start throwing my arms around and just jumping around and standing up and playing and just hitting it with anything I can ... and just ... the music just takes over, and I guess people can see that, so they think, 'Oh yeah, that's his passion, so we'll class him as a muso'. Which I'm happy to be classed as a muso, but yeah.

GT: But you're also a sporty person ...

Jake: Yeah, that's why I wouldn't just say I'm a muso.

GT: And do you think there are people ... that's the case for a lot of people? Like they'll classify them as a sporty person where in fact they might play music? How meaningful are the labels?

Jake: Yeah, um ... I don't know. Not really ... you don't get too many people that are really interested in sport that play music. I don't find ... like of course you'll get a few, but the majority will either be interested in sport or interested in music.

GT: Is there a tension between those groups?

Jake:	Not at all.
GT:	So kids don't get picked on if they ...
Jake:	No, no it's all good. It's actually really good as far as that goes. Like you're going to get kids that pick fights and stuff with anyone, but apart from that, it's really good, no one goes around 'You're a muso,' 'You're an idiot', 'You're a Goth ... look at you'.

Jake described how the labels had relevance and how they were also irrelevant. While he was happy to be known as a 'muso' he was more than this. His interest in sport broadened what it meant to be a muso. He was adamant, however, that school was a comfortable place to be regardless of whether you were muso, sporty, or Goth. I asked him to consider why students a this school did not pick on each other as was the case elsewhere. He commented:

Jake:	Yeah ... like other people you interview will probably say different things. I think, I don't know.
GT:	You don't know why that happens? Because I must say from my point of view, as an onlooker, it strikes me as a very tolerant place. Have I got that right?
Jake:	Yeah, yeah.
GT:	Kids seem to sort of not pick on each other?
Jake:	Yeah, I guess. Because we do have people that are a bit gay ... a bit unusual ... but I guess people just sort of accept it. And especially when you're in older age groups, when you're in younger age groups people will be like 'Oh yeah, you're a bit weird, so we'll just give you a hard time.' But as you get older, people just sort of mature and it becomes a lot easier to get on with people and everyone's sort of friends.

At one level, Jake's comments illustrate that kids at the top of the pecking order have little to resent. Along with (or perhaps because of) his good looks, his sporting abilities, and musical prowess, Jake was clearly someone others wanted to befriend. His casual style, quick smile, and quiet self-confidence put others at ease. He was popular with students and staff alike. He was also related to one of the senior members of staff. He experienced the school in a positive way and argued the benign nature of its subcultures. According to Jake, there were a few 'mingles' or fights, but these were not a significant part of the school. Students knew some students were 'nerds', but they were not referred to as such. This tolerance was a benchmark of maturity. Those who are a 'bit unusual' aren't seriously disadvantaged, particularly in senior years when everyone is mature enough to appreciate such difference. Yet his comment that others may 'say different things' hinted that his experience may not be universal. Certainly if by 'gay' Jake meant homosexual boys, there were those, even in senior years, who complained of harassment. (It is important to note in this context, that students did use 'gay' to mean unfashionable or conservative as well as homosexual.) Jake understood that 'nerds' were academic high achievers but this came at the cost of doing the extracurricular activities that for him stopped school becoming boring. In general terms, he believed that good results were a product of 'putting in the yards' of doing the work. He reiterated the dominant narrative at the school, everything was possible if students organised their time efficiently, planned their schedules, and did the work expected of them by teachers. Success was a product of effort rather than aptitude. However, Jake also hinted at a more skeptical view with his comment about 'genetics'.

Students believed Jake was a muso and he understood that he had earned this label through being see on stage and rehearsing at lunchtimes. Yet he illustrated how membership to one group was seen also to preclude membership of another group, in his case those who played sport. Being sporty and being a muso were not represented as compatible. Jake, makes particular reference to the teacher's comment that he couldn't be a 'real' muso if he was also good at sport. Yet in spite of this representation of 'musos', Jake who epitomised this subculture, illustrated the shifting nature of such labels, something he was aware of himself. He was happy to own the label 'muso', which for him related to passion and feeling about music rather than time spent playing, there was another side of him immersed in sport. The sporty Jake was less publicly identified but equally meaningful to him.

Being Middling

Like Jake, Ben, and Aaron were also deeply involved in the school music program, but cut a very different image around the school by comparison. They were commonly seen together and at first impression seemed less 'stand out' and charismatic. They were quieter and spent less time in the public gaze. Like Jake, they were in the final stages of Year 11 at the time of the interview and in a similar fashion, contemplating their final year of school. Ben wanted to study law and stated that this had been his ambition since he was seven years old. Aaron wanted to study engineering and because of his love of music, thought he may be able to combine both interests through doing 'courses to go into sound engineering and stage work.'

Apart from the official school bands, many students played, together in bands they had established for themselves and used the school premises for rehearsals. Some of these were beginning to perform publicly in clubs or hotels. In some cases, past students were involved in these bands. There seemed to be a hierarchy of talent at the school that was partly related to the age of students, the instruments they played, and their levels of musicianship. At the time of the study, Jake was in the band that was considered the most proficient and it was developing its own profile outside the school. Ben and Aaron were involved in another band, which was considered to have less status in these terms. Ben was a talented saxophonist and Aaron played electric guitar, an instrument not supported through the formal school curriculum.

> **GT:** Music — is it a really big part of your lives?
>
> **Ben:** Oh, yes, it's a good way to escape from schoolwork and stuff like that.
>
> **Aaron:** Good relaxation after school on Friday. Yes.
>
> **GT:** And do you play out of school, like are you in one of these bands that do pub circuits?
>
> **Ben:** Not yet.
>
> **GT:** Aspiring?
>
> **Ben:** Yes, aspiring. It's hard because we've got a bit of a mixture of instruments with a trumpet, a sax and a couple of guitars and that, so we're trying to find our styles. Still exploring at the moment. More jazz music and stuff. We're playing a few of the rock and roll songs we found work alright.
>
> **Aaron:** Like Elvis and stuff.
>
> **Ben:** It's fairly simple music.

For Ben and Aaron music was not described as a 'passion' and instead was represented as 'relaxation on a Friday' — a means of escaping the pressures of schoolwork. This became increasingly evident as they described the students who did well at school and situated themselves within the group for whom schoolwork was a high priority.

> As soon as it hits the end of Year 10, a lot of the students — there's a big change in their attitude towards the work, because they kind of think 'Oh, yeah, I'm going to have to get somewhere after school'. It's just not going to be my life, so they kind of change and want to do well to get to where they want to go. (Aaron)

They described how this had applied to about half of their year level and I asked if there was anything that distinguished this conscientious half from the other half.

> **Aaron:** I think girls are more conscientious probably about their work.
>
> **Ben:** Mature. I guess.

Aaron: I think in the end they do — yeah, they catch up.

GT: Now one of the things that I'd like to talk about are different groups of kids. Do you see that?

Ben: Oh, yes.

Aaron: It's quite noticeable.

Ben: In the school you know a lot of different groups — and outside of school you know there are sort of set groups. Sometimes they do mix, but there's a set group in many other schools I reckon.

GT: Can you tell me more about that.

Aaron: I'm lucky because I'm accepted into a diverse social group and friendship circles and stuff. I'm friendly like you guys, with Jack and the guys that enjoy music and stuff like that and like I'm also friendly with other kids, like Todd who enjoys sport, and footy and ... people like that.

Ben: You've sort of got your social groups. You've got your lower, middle, and high — not really low but you know ... I think I'm in the middle group and so if you're in the middle group you usually interact with both.

Aaron: Yes. You've got the best of both.

Ben: Go out and get drunk every Friday night and Saturday night and no, no, no.

Aaron: You wish.

Ben: No, you know — we're a bit more subtle in our ways, the middle group.

Aaron: The middle group — everything in moderation.

Ben: Has a bit to drink but not too much and there's a lot of drugs and stuff in that high group you know, but they're all good guys still.

Aaron: I don't think any of them have been in serious trouble before.

Ben: Yes, they're not like ... they couldn't get arrested. They're not into that serious stuff, but as far as I've encountered so far, it's not really serious stuff that they do.

GT: And the low group?

Aaron: Probably never got drunk, they're more reserved, more focused, it's alright, they're good guys as well. Probably wanting to do a bit better in their academic work and stuff.

GT: And do the girls fit in both groups and get into their own groups as well or have they added a different perspective?

Ben: They sort of fit into the group and they also get into their own group as well. Within that — it's like a simple one — you've got all these different groups, musos and sports people and that.

GT:	Tell me more.
Ben:	We play in a band together — so we've got groups like that you know and we talk about music together and that, yet we can go out and play footy as well. We got out and talk to the guys that play footy, rugby, and so we sort of — there's people that are focused on sport, and you get to know different people that fit into different groups.
GT:	And they're all happy with each other?
Aaron:	Yes. You mean within each group and stuff or between groups.
GT:	Between groups, yes.
Aaron:	There can be fights, definitely, at times. Often you get like they're protagonists, who kind of often want to start fights and stuff like that, but …
Ben:	There's a few people always fighting, especially with the low groups like they feel bad you know. There's always going to be a couple, but basically yes, the middle group gets along with both so …

While Ben and Aaron fleetingly refer to groups such as the musos and sporty kids, they choose to emphasise status levels instead. In their terms, the low group concentrates on school work while the high group is associated with drugs and alcohol. In the middle they do things 'in moderation' and 'have the best of both'. Ben and Aaron are quick to qualify their description of the high group: they're good guys and not the type to get arrested. Unlike their description of students at other schools, these students are recreational rather than serious drinkers, smokers, or drug takers. There is respect for the 'coolness' of the high group implied in Aaron's 'you wish' response to Ben's joking description of his drinking on the weekend. These boys recognise the social sacrifice implicit in their membership of the middle group. Their comments remained fuzzy around the issue of fighting — this existed through certain 'protagonists' but it was something they did not wish to elaborate.

These somewhat veiled comments characterised the flavour of this interview — a sense of hinting at issues but not wishing to expand. Again, as an interviewer, you can only guess at whether this is an appropriate interpretation and if so, the reasons. Were they withholding specific information or simply not expressing themselves in expansive ways, arguably typical of boys their age. Were they hinting at drugs and alcohol as a means of indicating that they were 'in the loop' with the 'cool' kids? Or perhaps they were pulling their punches for fear of getting kids into trouble or shedding poor light on the school? These boys also differentiated between girls and boys. In their terms, girls are 'conscientious' and 'more mature' — in the end they 'catch up' with the boys. Again they don't elaborate further on these comments, which imply a range of common-sense understandings about girls doing well through hard work rather than capability. In a similar way, they do not elaborate how girls are part of the groups they describe, but also have their own groups and 'perspectives'.

Ben spoke with a heavy South African accent. He told me that he came from Johannesburg. The boys agreed that there were many South Africans in Australia and recognised some at their school. They described this group as moving between schools.

Ben: There's a couple [South Africans] who have left over the years.

Aaron: Yes, Barry he went to [elite independent school], didn't he?

GT: And is there a lot of movement between private schools and here?

Ben: Some of the people, I don't know left for [elite independent school] like last year ...

Aaron: Nick left and went to Melbourne High [select-entry government boys school] I suppose, I don't know, maybe they ...

GT: Melbourne High — that's not a private school.

Ben: It's not private, but I think that it's rated as the top government school.

Aaron: Because his brother did really well. He got like 99 in his score, so I think they would have accepted him.

Ben: I find that actually, there's more people shifting from public to private schools than there are from private to public. Maybe, because there's only one guy that I can think of right now that came from a private school, so yes, so I don't know. I think there's more movement.

This sequence illustrates the awareness of school status and choice amongst students. It also illustrates the 'fuzziness' that surrounds entry into certain government schools. Melbourne High is the select government school. Unlike Leafy Suburbs College, there is no assumption that siblings can enter automatically. The sequence may also illustrate the significance attached to such school choice within the South African community. As with the Russian community, many South African immigrants are also Jewish. Both Aaron and Ben are Jewish and this became evident during the interview when Aaron mentioned that he had attended a Jewish primary school. Aaron and Ben agreed that being Jewish provided a focus within the school community.

Aaron: I think it's like an underlying thing, like all the Jewish people know who they are and like everyone knows who you are and stuff if you're Jewish. But I don't think it's one of the main aspects which determines your social groups and stuff, but it is an underlying thing like. You know who is Jewish and probably because of your parents or shul obviously you have lives outside school where you — like religious lives or whatever. I mean I'm not religious but I go to shul occasionally which is like synagogue which is like a Jewish church or whatever and yes you meet people. And like your parents I don't know — often Jewish parents know a bit of everything. They know everything, I don't know, for some reason.

Ben: When you've got like Jewish festivals and that, sometimes you talk about it but it's not really that big. When you've got stuff like Bar Mitzvahs and that you know, it comes into it a bit there, but not very often I don't think. It's not just Jewish people but I'm saying it's like, I mean you wouldn't talk about what you're eating and that, because they wouldn't know, or sometimes they do but they don't understand really what you're talking about.

GT: Oh, okay, but it's not a separate social scene?

Aaron: No, I wouldn't say that but a lot of people they are, like people like Ingrid and stuff they're often involved in outside Jewish youth movements.

Ben: They go on camps, just like get all Jewish people together. They're [Jewish youth groups] all the same just varying degrees of how religious they are. They just go on camps and have fun and you know organise footy matches, fun footy matches and stuff.

GT: And are you guys involved in that?

Aaron: I would be but I work on a Saturday and that's when they hold their meetings.

Ben: I played footy once. Yes, I've been to a couple of meetings, but you know they hold their camps and I usually go away around then, like around Christmas time, so I usually go away around then so I don't usually go on the camps but I've got a couple of friends who go so I've been a couple of times.

GT: But it's comfortable being Jewish at the school isn't it?

Ben: Yes, yes.

GT: In some schools there are problems.

Aaron: Often you get, like when you're playing around with people and stuff, often they'll say, 'Oh, are you Jewish?' or something, but not in a … you'd never get it in a direct like, racist kind of way.

GT: But you feel there's an undercurrent there?

Ben: Yes, but they don't mean it. Like a lot of people can say stuff, but they don't know what they're saying, but it doesn't matter to us you know. Because we know their intentions and I know personally — no one has ever said anything to me with bad intentions or anything like so …

GT: They use the word without meaning …

Ben: Yes, they're just having a bit of fun. You know some people poke fun.

Aaron:	Yes, I often get it because I'm South African so …
GT:	What do they say about being South African?
Aaron:	Nothing, I just often get my accent, just sometimes people mock your accent. The teachers.
Ben:	Yes. Mr White.
Aaron:	Yes, Mr White and Mr Black. He was horrible. Cricket or something.
Ben:	When South African went out of the World Cup, Aaron copped a bit in the end.
Aaron:	Yes, but mainly in sport mostly. Definitely mainly sport. If something happens to the South African sporting team, then often I get it, but it's never in like bad taste, I don't think.

In this section of the interview, Aaron and Ben signal three important aspects of identification for them. Their Jewishness; in the case of Aaron, coming from South Africa; and the link between masculinity and sport. Jewishness was part of these boys' identities. It was an undercurrent that may not have cut across their being in the middle social group, but it certainly flavoured who they were and their interactions with other students. They had access to a Jewish community at the school and outside it through shul and related youth organisations. In their case, it was something that they dipped into. Relative to other students they had described, they were not as committed to such organisations. While non-Jewish students participated in some Jewish traditions such as Bar Mitzvahs, these boys felt there were aspects of their religion that were not commonly understood. Implied in their comments was the fact that the naming of students as Jewish may also cause discomfort. They differentiated this from overt racism. Here, there was slippage between being South African and Jewish. But in both cases, comments are attributed to 'having fun', 'bad taste', or using words without 'bad intention'. It is in this context that these students mention sport in relation to banter between themselves and members of staff. Sport is a significant issue in Australia and with regard to those from ethnic minorities it comes up as a means of testing national loyalties. With regard to events such as the Olympics, international soccer competitions and cricket, 'foreigners' are put to the test, particularly when Australia is involved in direct competition with nations such as South Africa, a country of origin for immigrants. This sequence illustrates the significance of sport within school communities and how it can serve as a common interest between male staff and boys. I have argued elsewhere that girls may not have access to equivalent forms of camaraderie (Tsolidis 1986). In this context, however, these boys hint at the negative side of such common interest. In the case of Mr White and Mr Gray, however, this may have been particularly overt given their reputation within the school. Other students and some members of staff had highlighted their authoritarian and conservative attitude, in general, and in relation to their interactions with students. They were close friends and unpopular with some students and staff. One member of staff had described Mr White to me as 'that pain in the arse'. She was particularly hostile to him because of his authoritarian attitudes to students. Perhaps in this instance, Ben and Aaron's interpretation of his comments as indicating no ill intention was overly generous.

Ben and Aaron were positive about Leafy Suburbs College and felt that what it had to offer was superior to other schools, including some independent schools.

Ben:	I think the social structures are more subtle here than at a lot of other schools, you know like. There's always a chance of people you know, like there is a distinction between the groups, but you know it's not as bad as some other places I reckon. You've always got the people that tease and that, but I mean I think it's better than a lot of other schools.
GT:	Why do you think that it's better?
Ben:	Because a lot of people get along. There's only a few people that don't get along out of a class of 190 or something like that.
GT:	And what are they like — the kids that don't along?
Ben:	Well, like one guy just had honey poured in his locker and there was all these ants all over it and so …
GT:	So what was it about him that …
Ben:	He's very eccentric and very …
Aaron:	He's got to be able to cause trouble often. I'd say he brings it on himself a lot of the time.
Ben:	Yes, he brings it on himself because it's not a matter of the high group picking on the low group there, it's just …
Aaron:	Everyone picking on him because he's a …
Ben:	It brings everyone together.
Aaron:	Kind of like a unified effort.
Ben:	Yes, last week he got superglue put in his locker, um honey poured in his locker. I think they were all Year 12s that did it. He's not very popular even though he thinks he is.
Aaron:	Yes, that's one of the main things. He thinks he's this high and mighty guy, but he kind of tries too hard sometimes.

Ben and Aaron suggest that a sense of community exists at Leafy Suburbs College. On the whole, the social groups that exist are benign. While there is risk-taking behaviour within the 'high' group, this is not extreme. Students who do get picked on are few and 'bring it on themselves'. They nominate one such student out of close to two hundred.

Ben and Aaron are students with high aspirations. Their interest in music compliments a range of other activities including sport, part-time work, and activities outside the school associated with the Jewish community. While music is important to their sense of self, it does not dominate. In the interview itself, it takes up very little time. Jake, on the other hand, had more subdued academic aspirations; carpentry and alternative medicine do not require the same end-of-school results as law and engineering. Within the school, it is his musicianship that focuses attention. Another contrasting aspect between these students relates to their ethnic identity. Aaron and Ben identify as Jewish and discuss this in relative detail. Jake, on the other hand, makes little of his Greek background. Jake is happy to describe his background as half Greek, discuss his trips to Greece, and his limited capacity to communicate with grandparents for whom Greek is still the main language spoken. There is no hint of wishing to conceal this aspect of his identity. On the other hand, there is no sense of wanting to give it any prominence. Jake, Ben, and Aaron are all avid and talented musicians who spend a great deal of time playing music in bands inside and outside schools. All three were all strongly identified as 'musos' within the school. Yet only Aaron aims to integrate his love of music with his future career, and this in a tenuous way. He wants to become an engineer and possibly, given his interest in music, do this in relation to stage and sound engineering.

While there was an extensive music program at Leafy Suburbs College, the students who played classical music were not identified as 'musos' by staff and students involved in the study. This label was reserved for those students involved in bands, quartets, or trios that performed jazz music and who stood out as soloists within these contexts. They were students who had some standing as musicians. Commonly, these students were also involved in other aspects of school life, including in leadership roles. However, being a 'muso' meant also being a little bit different; there was something of the avant-garde about these students — students who were trendsetters. In the next chapter, an interview with a further two 'musos' will be discussed. While this aspect of their identities was foremost in other students' descriptions of them, it was evident that this was not the only thing that made them 'awesome', and therefore, students others felt I must include in the study.

Chapter 9

Synthesising Selves

There was a great deal of music happening at the school. Yet it was clear that for some students, music was relaxation, something that helped them cope with the demands of a rigorous academic program, while for others it anchored an identity in ways that went beyond the norm. In the case of Sebastian and Julian, music was central to what appeared as a highly choreographed sense of self that revolved around being different. Yet these were not your death-obsessed Goths, angry heavy metal fans, or your self-absorbed disco 'clubbers'. Instead, these boys and their circle of friends personified a type of cultivated quietness and muted hyperinvolvement in the school. They appeared at the school concerts in an array of ensembles; they were there at the art exhibitions but always quiet, unassuming and yet very noticeable. To a great extent, this was due to the extreme hairstyles these students chose (dread locks, a head full of thinly plaited hair). In the case of Sebastian and Julian, the fact that they were twins and unusually talented in a range of fields also made them stand out. This was talent in contradistinction to diligence, which meant that despite high achievement, they would never be mistaken for 'nerds'. These students did their work, but did not rely on hard work to achieve. Further to this, they toed the line, but understood this as a choice rather than a battle with authority. Their coupling of extreme hairstyles with school uniform seemed to represent a compromise — a give and take between the school and themselves.

Sebastian and Julian had an aura about them, especially with the younger students who spoke of them almost in hushed tones. They were students others thought I 'had to' interview, and were strongly identified as musos. At the beginning of the study, I had assumed it would be too difficult to involve students who were in their final year of schooling because of the pressures of exams. As it turned out, these students had completed their exams and were most amenable to being interviewed. At the time of the interview they were in the process of selecting tertiary courses for which they would apply. They returned to the school for the interview, but were not in school uniform and their choice of clothing added a dimension to their personalities that had not been obvious with many other interviewees. Their outfits were a pastiche of old and new, colourful hats, waistcoats, and footwear that on other students may have seemed gauche, but in their case, given their quiet and unassuming personas, appeared instead to evidence their creativity. Being identical twins was an important part of their identities. They finished each other's sentences and in many ways it was like interviewing one rather than two people. We began the interview with an exploration of the courses they hoped to enter the following year. They had studied music in their final year of schooling and like Jake, Ben, and Aaron were not planning to continue with music in their tertiary studies. They had also studied graphic arts and were hoping to continue this interest, possibly related to music in some way. These boys were extremely articulate and thoughtful. They made mention of having studied English Literature in Year 12 and how this had altered their thinking. They explained their reasons for not continuing their music studies:

Sebastian: No, because we've heard all these horror stories about how hard a muso's life is, although if we do get into a course this year we're going to defer for a year and then see, have a crack at making it in the music industry and you know ...

Julian: Yes, or not so much, we're just going to try and get some stuff recorded and fiddle around and see what happens, see if it works, and if it works maybe keep going with it on the side, because I mean whatever happens with it, we're definitely still going to be doing music as a hobby or whatever just because we enjoy it so much and you know we've got each other. We can kind of jam with each other and all of that.

Sebastian: Yes, that's really good.

GT: What do you play?

Sebastian: Bits of everything. Double bass.

Julian: Bass, guitar, cello, French horn. Between us we have a small orchestra.

Sebastian: A little bit of piano.

Julian:	We both play guitar. Sebastian can fiddle his way through bass. I can fiddle my way through drums. I play the cello, he plays the French horn, so we've got everything.
GT:	So what makes a muso's life too hard?
Sebastian:	Well, it's hard to make enough money, get enough solid employment solely as a muso to kind of subsist within …
Julian:	There's no constant employment, there's no constant money source. You've got to …
Sebastian:	Unless you get a residency or something which is like a stable gig every month or so and you get really lucky and get famous and discovered and then supposedly the money just rolls in, but either way, it's supposedly a very stressful lifestyle, constant demands.

Like Jake, Aaron, and Ben, Sebastian and Julian argued that music could not provide the income that was necessary for a comfortable and stable lifestyle. However, they seemed more reluctant than others to relegate it to the purely recreational. They wanted to experiment with 'making it in the industry' in the year between finishing school and beginning tertiary study. Jake argued that music was unlikely to provide the income necessary for his future lifestyle that involved costly pursuits such as skiing. Sebastian and Julian were concerned about stress and this is a theme that they return to throughout the interview. In this context, the music industry is stressful because the demands are too great and because the income is unpredictable.

Julian and Sebastian stated that they were extremely interested in the issue of student subcultures. They had spent time talking to each other about the topic quite independently of the interview and their interest in music prompted their description of these subcultures in relation to music styles and preferences.

GT:	Do you recognise subgroups in the school?
Julian:	Oh, God yes. Sebastian is very good at this. This is a bit of a …
Sebastian:	I wouldn't say I'm good at it, I'd say I just like to rant about it a lot.
GT:	Please rant. This is what I'm really interested in.
Julian:	You've picked the right person.
Sebastian:	Oh, God yes, I don't know how much of this is going to be accurate because I'm shockingly biased. There's always groups. They can be really easily identified in the earlier years, they can be easily identified and are often very closed, you know in certain groups there will be the unpopular children, they're generally — they are usually together and for some reason can be seen playing four-square. And there's the trendy kids which you know they

	— it's hard, the trendy kids thing doesn't quite kick in in the earlier years, but as it goes further up in the school it becomes more easy to see the trendy kids. They also hang about in large groups — similar fashions — you know, similar lifestyle which was probably what led them to group together and all that sort of stuff, and then there's the — I tend to link a lot of this stuff to music so …
Julian:	Yeah, music and fashion, kind of are key things in the formation of these groups, or in kind of what identifies them in those groups.
Sebastian:	If not a cause then it's a symptom, because it's similar music tastes and similar fashion sense that leads them to be in the same groups, so there's the people that listen to pop music and music that is popular, not necessarily the same thing, here we go …
GT:	Ok, give me an example.
Sebastian:	There's the Rap R&B [rhythm and blues] and Soul crowd that we have at this school.
Julian:	They're often kind of ethnic minorities, for no reason that I can identify.
Sebastian:	It may be a bit of a stereotype or generalisation, but like most, it does seem to be truth in there, and there is a definite crowd about that.
Julian:	That kind of gang type of stereotype.
GT:	Is that what people call the 'wogs'?
Sebastian:	That's part of it yes, yes. That's just one because there's also the Russians, the Kurds, the Turks and it just goes …
Julian:	And they've each got their own kind of cultural stereotypes that they either rebel against or kind of embody, either for entertainment or unconsciously.
Sebastian:	With that group there's a gang element in it to a certain extent, banding together and all of that, partly because of the music which does, a lot of hip hop and rap does, promote or glorify the gang lifestyle, that you know band together with those who are like-minded or similarly disadvantaged to kind of make a changing situation. It starts off a positive thing — but I mean it seems a positive thing, but for some reason it doesn't work out that way. But then communism seems like a positive thing and that's never worked here.
Julian:	Great idea.
Sebastian:	They wear plastic clothes.

Sebastian and Julian loved the topic under discussion, loved to talk, and in this way were the interviewer's dream 'subjects'. In their comments here, they identify relevant music and then the subgroups that they associate with the music. In their exploration of these topics I felt that I was listening to them relate a range of theory to their own experience — making sense of their own school via deconstructive methods perhaps acquired in the English Literature classroom. Here, 'ethnic minority' kids are 'gangsters'. Theirs is a community that comes out of wanting to change a disadvantage. This is both 'stereotype' and truth. And like communism it begins with the best intentions but never works. They return regularly to the idea of stereotypes and the possibility that these can be escaped.

Sebastian: Everyone really hates being classified because I mean even me, myself, I really don't like being classified at a certain level, but at the same time I realise there's no way I'm really going to escape.

Julian: Nobody likes to be classified, but there's no way ...

Sebastian: They don't like the idea that they can be pigeonholed.

Julian: You can look at someone and say 'Oh, that person is a trendy and therefore they will listen to, you know pop artists, Britney Speares, Pink', all that sort of stuff. You know they could listen to something like say Germaine and the Cat Empire which wouldn't be associated with that, but you know it's a generalisation, you can never know. You can't look at someone and say 'Oh, that person is a trendy' and automatically know everything about them because they're always going to have something that doesn't fit into that particular group.

GT: But you can name the group doing it? So what is it?

Sebastian: With great relish — I love it.

GT: So what are some of the other groups? We've had the ... what was the first one?

Sebastian: There's the trendies, then there's the R&Bs, Soul crowd.

Julian: Gangsters.

Sebastian: Often there's a bit of relation between the two because ...

Julian: There is in England.

Sebastian: Yes, hip hop and R&B are becoming more popular as they're moving more towards the mainstream and as a result these two groups have been intermingling somewhat.

Julian: And then there's the alternatives, which disavow everything to do with those two previous groups.

Sebastian: The trendy alternatives and the not-trendy alternatives. It just gets into insane levels.

Julian: The trendy alternatives are the ones who, here we go, how can I do this without ...

Sebastian: Proclaim individuality en masse, kind of as a group.

Julian: 'We are all individuals.' Individuality as a collective. Then there's the non-trendy alternatives who hate the trendies because they're trendy, hate the alternatives because they have become trendy as well, because they have some success. They're the ones who have little sense of belonging and that's what identifies, that's what defines their group and those who they hang around with.

Sebastian: So a lot of the groups really don't mix because they kind of look and think 'Ok, that's a bit scary', or they're a bit too different, so maybe uncomfortable. It's because they don't have, I don't know, that shared experience that defines these groups, they don't understand why these things happen, why they have those certain types of people, different collective subjectivities. So you'll see, it's almost, it's sort of racism, it's just an ignorance and a mistrust based on that ignorance and it's often based on an outward appearance, little more than that.

Julian: Like you see someone with a four-feet-high green mohawk and you automatically think — alright that guy is a punk, is a criminal, he would be violent, disrespectful of any sort of authority, but for all you know he could have a nice job and he gives his money to his mum.

In this sequence, rather than simply describe the subcultures, Julian and Sebastian explain why subcultures form and why they are both valid and a generalisation. Some subcultures are a 'collective subjectivity'. They provide a much-needed sense of belonging for those who experience alienation. For other subcultures, however, being different becomes a massified and manufactured alternative. Sebastian and Julian were concerned with how difference is consumed and therefore becomes mainstream. They also understood the danger implicit in creating categories. In their own comments they provided characterisation of the categories coupled with a running commentary of how stereotypes needed to be challenged — a punk can be someone who gives money to his mum.

GT: So do you identify with any of the groups you've nominated?

Sebastian: I don't know. We jump back and forth between them.

Julian: And kind of alter our behaviour and appearance to kind of think with that group, but we can anyway. We like to think we do.

GT: And how do you think they see you, as you present yourselves?

Sebastian: I have a bit of a problem with that because the image I'm trying to present is always going to be completely different to the image that other people are going to get of me, and so it's always a bit of a problem kind of trying to — because if you let it get to you too much you end up synthesising yourself to the stage where you can't, where you're kind of uncomfortable in any

Julian:	given situation because you're too preoccupied with it — so you've just got to kind of work out what it is about this group that you like and if you don't like it, change it, or if you can't change it, live with it.
Julian:	And just in doing that, you all drift into these groups, find people who are similar and you've just got to. I think the groups then — they don't really have to limit you although for a lot of people they seem to. All you've got to do is kind of realise, oh yeah, there are so many social groups and if I really don't like being in one I'm going to walk out of one straight into another and I think, yeah, hating someone just because of their particular social group or music taste or whatever is pointless because …
Julian:	But then so is hating someone because their sink hole is different …
GT:	So are these groups equal in the food chain?
Sebastian:	Well, to themselves they are. Each of the groups thinks that they're top dogs and kind of thinks all the others are really slightly below them, second-class citizens, but objectively the rest of the world really doesn't care that much about what these particular groups are thinking so …

Synthesising self — for these boys, the aim is to avoid being identified with one particular group. Instead, they jump between these groups, remaining comfortable with themselves by recognising that they cannot control the ways others see them and cannot remain totally outside the box. Their solution is to remain fluid, eclectic, and tolerant. Power is not an issue because every group thinks it is the best one and when all is said and done, the rest of the world does not really care.

Sebastian:	I would say that the trendies and the pop alternatives would be the two largest groups, they're the two largest groups here. The pop alternative is catching up pretty quickly because there's been a movement towards that just because of the lifestyle, just slightly …
Julian:	Revival of the punk and all of that.
Sebastian:	Yes, disrespect for authority without going too far out of line to get yourself ostracised.
Julian:	So it's like claiming yourself to be an exile, which on the face of it does seem like it shouldn't work but it has so far.
GT:	And do you link authority or power with numbers?
Julian:	Not really since …
Sebastian:	Oh, to a certain extent, with a lot of the groups. Even the ones that I think of being the powerful groups base themselves on disrespecting power. You know you think, 'Oh, teenagers in a group, scary', just because there's a large group of kids there. I mean even me, I'm afraid to walk the streets at night.

Julian: Trendies will rebel against their parents, alternatives will rebel against everybody, rebel against the law, stereotypes ...

Sebastian: I mean we know that, ourselves we are stereotyped and we enjoy it.

GT: Why are you stereotypes?

Sebastian: Oh, because we can acknowledge these things inside ourselves.

Julian: I mean I know that I, I mean we've got the rather odd clothing, the dreadlocks, all of that kind of stuff, but we're definitely, I mean even if it's just the image we project, there's not much of a chance of being able to project yourself as something that hasn't been done before because any kind of assumptions that people are going to make about you are based on previous experience anyway.

Sebastian: We can recognise these things in other people and ourselves, and also we can say, oh, I dress differently, I have odd hair you know, I listen to such and such a music style, so I could probably be classified as such and such you know. We'd be sort of bending the alternatives.

Again, in this exchange, Julian and Sebastian illustrate their reflective natures. They understand that they are stereotypes, but by projecting a stereotype knowingly, they are somehow also challenging the predictability of putting people in pigeon boxes. Because of knowing — that people stereotype and that there is no possibility of doing something that hasn't been done before — projecting a stereotype becomes enjoyable because it epitomises irony. As Julian comments, presenting yourself as an exile does work, to a great extent. Projecting yourself as an exile also works because it stays within safe boundaries. After all, these students are choosing exile rather than dealing with its imposition; because of this, they can also choose not to be exiles. The North African refugee students in neighbouring housing estates, on the other hand, do not need to project themselves as exiles. This has been done on their behalf. Nor can they slip out of this exile in such easy ways.

GT: But none of that seems, I mean as an outsider I wouldn't have thought about it like you. I think the kids seem to get along alright with each other.

Sebastian: I think a lot of that would be the uniform because I mean at school you don't have that kind of — the obvious visual division in the clothes, or the hair or anything like that. At Alternative College — all our friends who go to Alternative — there's not much interaction between the groups, like the drama and performing arts students here only ever talk to the performing arts students and occasionally the musos and other artists. There, there are definite divisions if only because they take the same kind of subjects, but also with the lack of uniform and the ability to assert yourself as belonging to any of those particular groups with an appearance or whatever.

Julian: In the school situation you pretty much have to be there. If you're there then you are — yeah, it's not like you have any choice in the matter. You're in the class with whoever. You don't have much choice, therefore you sort of have to get it on. If you don't, then, you will probably find somewhere else to go. It's happened before — people who aren't getting along with anybody or you know getting along with so few people as to make it unbearable, well generally you have to do something else.

Sebastian: Oh well, it's the situation. The fact that you're thrown into the same lot, because you're all in the same kind of environment, undergoing the same experience, it's that shared experience thing again. Now that we've finished school, we won't see so many of these people again just because they're not in the groups that we associate with — and kind of the only shared experience we have is the school, so all these groups that I've identified are technically subgroups to the larger student body.

Julian: The fact that we are students or young people, or — because these groups overlap a lot and also overlap with other types of groups, male/female, black hair/red hair, all of that kind of stuff, so yeah, it's all a bit confusing really.

For Julian and Sebastian, it is not a case of harmony existing at Leafy Suburbs College. Instead, they argue that the strict uniform policy camouflages difference and provides a sense of a shared identity. Students have to be together, they have school in common. The experience of the school becomes the overarching commonality. Once school is over, they will only see those they associate with by choice rather than circumstance. They compare this situation to Alternative College, the neighbourhood school that is commonly juxtaposed to Leafy Suburbs College. This is also a government school, but one that is not conservative. There is no uniform and the school has a reputation for less discipline, being more student centred, and valuing the creative arts. Students can be themselves, learn in their own way. Students who leave Leafy Suburbs College tend to go to Alternative College. Because of the more liberal atmosphere at this school, Sebastian and Julian argue that it is possible to complicate the categories. Subject selection crosses boundaries with dress sense, for example, so that students have more identity choices. In this sequence, Julian and Sebastian introduce the significance of shared experience and elaborate on it further as the interview continues.

GT: I think it's very interesting. Is there anything we haven't mentioned, gender, for example, is that an issue do you think?

Sebastian: To some extent yeah, sometimes, not so much now as it was — it might have been ten years ago or something, but yes, it's background, it's all subject to the socioeconomic background and all that sort of stuff. Also it's a comfort thing, like minorities will often sit together because of shared experience

— it's another group — and with that comes certain mind-sets or you know things like — cultural idiosyncrasies that lead them towards certain things like a lot of minorities often turn to the R&B hip hop group because it expresses what they kind of — the message of solidarity and the minority holding out against this larger force.

Julian: I mean the reasons are pretty much the same whatever form it takes — whether it's joining youth groups or a gang, because even the alternative punk crowd — they do that because they have you know certain things about them that make them do that. Like they may have rich stuffy parents which leads them to the kind of thing like, 'I don't want to be anything like my parents', so they dress trashily and offensively and listen to loud music and all that sort of stuff.

Sebastian: We hang out with the people that we hang out with because we can identify with them and because we do have that shared experience with them.

Julian: Can I just rant about punk cultures more? The trendy punk, the pop alt. thing has gradually come about because people who don't have this inherent, you know this unpleasant condition — which is where punk has originally come from — it would lead them to punk but still — like in the sixties and fifties in England, bad home life and all that sort of stuff that would lead them to that punk lifestyle, which if they don't have that, but they still like the look of it. They get the sort of watered-down combination of the two, they synthesise it, so that's how you get the thing between the pop alt. and the true alternative but it's um …

Sebastian: True alternative which in itself is difficult. Alternative is a really bad word, the same as success is a really bad word.

Julian: You can't really say anything with any certainty because it's all subjective for one thing. This is what literature has done for us. We did literature as a subject …

GT: Oh, I can tell.

Sebastian: Oh, it's because we've got — a teenager these days has so much there.

Julian: We've got independence, we've got communication, we've got mobile phones, we can have jobs, make money.

GT: You've also got more to cannibalise. I find it fascinating that you're so interested in the seventies you know, retro. It's fascinating, and what you see now are fashions that are this generation's versions of seventies' fashion.

Sebastian: And now we're going op shopping for the kind of stuff that you went to op shops not to buy.

Julian: That's probably what makes it so difficult because you know there's nothing really new about it, it's just the next generation's take on it, what they choose to do with it.

For these students, literature had taught them that there is no single take on reality. Everyone is 'subjective' and because of this, both 'alternative' and 'success' are bad words. Yet in their comments they seem to distinguish something that could be gleaned as authentic. There are those whose dress and music reflect experiences of harshness, the 'real' punks and those who imitate punk style without these experiences. Similarly, there are those who lived the seventies and those like Julian and Sebastian who try to find the seventies in opportunity shops. The caveat here, however, is that they go shopping for the things my generation would not have worn. In this way, straightforward mimicry is avoided and instead they continue performing the exile through synthesis.

GT: Would you recommend me interviewing anyone? Like your friends or enemies?

Sebastian: That's a difficult ... I mean anyone who actually thinks about this is going to have a lot to say, it's just whether you can get them thinking about it is the only thing. Don't interview too many Lit students because we're all biased.

Julian: I mean by the fact that we do Literature ourselves yes. I don't want to give names just because I feel uncomfortable.

GT: No, that's fine.

Sebastian: Having to kind of volunteer people — or not so much that, as having to say I think that person is a good example of such and such, you should talk to them, although if you walk up to anyone in a plastic tracksuit they would probably have something to say about ...

Julian: You're shocking!

Sebastian: I know, I know.

Julian: He's got an incredibly biased and dismissive view of everything.

Sebastian: Yeah, I know I'm very judgmental about stuff in general.

Julian and Sebastian declined nominating other students who I should interview. They did not want the responsibility of placing real people into the boxes they had created. They had learned the power of the word in literature and to 'give names' created discomfort. Yet they had strong opinions and resolved this tension by castigating themselves for being 'dismissive' and 'judgmental'. The comment about the 'plastic tracksuit' closes the circle opened at the beginning of the interview. It was the 'gangster' kids, those often referred to as 'wogs', who wore these outfits and were being named by not being named.

GT: Do you want to say anything that you haven't felt free to?

Sebastian: No, this has been good. I've had the chance to get a good rant — although recently my views have become a lot more tempered just because I've been able recently to look at myself. Up until recently you know I've been a hardcore punk. Nowadays I find just the fact that I used to call myself artful punk very easy, but yeah …

GT: What's made the change? Is it age?

Sebastian: Increased self-awareness I think. I look at myself more and I realise that the things I'm doing, I can laugh at them.

Julian: And look at himself as kind of his place in the rest of the world and the people around him.

Sebastian: That's partly what allows us to jump between some groups, because we can.

Julian: And I mean we've got each other. We can bounce ideas off each other like we have this same discussion …

Sebastian: This is what we talk about in coffee shops with all our other bohemian friends without shoes.

Julian: That's the stereotype and the shared subjectivity again.

Sebastian: I always make snide jokes about, it but while I'm talking about something dismissively I'll also …

Julian: Actually I tend to kind of dismiss my own viewpoint as well because you know, anything he says is meaningless as well. It's incredibly personal. I find all of these groups equally ridiculous. I find that the fact that humanity has evolved fashion, just the craziest thing — I mean how does that happen? How do people who used to use rocks to break open fruit to eat evolve saying certain clothes are better than others.

Sebastian: Or even that one thing looks better than another. How does that happen?

Julian: What does this bloke in Paris have to do with it and how did he get any authority to say this?

GT: Why do we give him the authority and everybody decides to wear these fashions?

Julian: It's a very odd thing, but I suppose if you enjoy it and if you want to do it, it's all good. I've got an opposite viewpoint to what he has, possibly just because he's so strong. I kind of reckon that as long as you're enjoying yourself, or as long as you're okay with it, then you keep on doing it.

For these boys, self-awareness had liberated them from the game of wanting to be different by naming themselves as such. Yet there was a strong understanding of this as a contradictory location. There is reference here to their 'bohemian' friends who wear no shoes and with whom they spend time in cafés.

By belonging to this group there is still belonging — a shared identity built on rejecting the very thing they criticise — projecting an en masse identity. Yet there was a clear understanding of this in itself being a contradictory location — of being guilty of the very things they criticised. Julian and Sebastian exhibited the same reflexivity with regard to naming others as more or less trendy. Through comments about 'plastic clothes', they were indicating their estimation of the worth of this style, yet there was also self-censure. Not willing to name the people who wore the 'plastic clothes' allowed them to maintain an integrity they valued. Theirs was a sense of no escape. No matter how you wanted to project yourself, others ultimately had control of how you would be understood. Each resolved this differently. For Julian it was a matter of pleasing yourself — if it feels good, do it. Sebastian, on the other hand, remains relatively perplexed and angry by the authority others have over him in this process. Julian explains his stance as a relative lack of strength. Sebastian, on the other hand, states that they jump between categories because they can and in this way emphasises their agency.

Unlike other students, Julian and Sebastian had completed school at the time of the interview. Perhaps this brought to the interview a perspective that put schooling very much in hindsight. Nonetheless, they were unusual students. More so than others interviewed, they seemed to epitomise successful adaptation to liquid modernity by understanding the disadvantages of durable identities. Here were students whose identifications were premised on shape shifting (Pollock 1997).

Julian and Sebastian were high academic achievers; however, they did not aspire to prestigious university courses such as law and medicine. Instead, they wanted to be involved in creative fields that allow them to extend their interest in graphics and possibly relate this to music as well. They were celebrating the end of a high-pressured period which included exams and course selection. This involved a range of interviews at universities where they had lodged applications. The end of school was their opportunity to relax and to apply for 'teenagey' employment before continuing their studies. During this period, they also anticipated continuing and expanding an existing interest with a Web-based music program they had developed with friends. This had commercial potential and while they downplayed its significance, it seemed to hold great significance in how they were shaping their futures. These were the sort of young people who humbled (or perhaps intimidated) my generation.

Here, a number of students who were identified as musos have been considered in some depth. Jake, Ben, Aaron, Sebastian, and Julian indicated that music was central to their lives. Each also had alternative aspects to their identities, but within the school, it seemed to others that a major aspect of who they were was linked to music. This needs to be seen in the context of a school where music had a significant presence. Leafy Suburbs College was known for its music program, which extended beyond the formal curriculum through a wide range of extracurricula activities.

There is evidence that extracurricula activities such as music assist with school engagement. There is also evidence that such engagement is important for academic success and is, in turn, linked to high socioeconomic status and parents with professional backgrounds. Achieving in nonacademic programs develops self-esteem and leadership qualities. In Australia, independent school students benefit the most from school programs that offer a variety of extracurricula activities and government school students benefit least (Fullerton 2002). Leafy Suburbs College offers a range of extracurricula programs including a wide range of sports, theatre, debating, leadership programs, camps, student exchanges to various countries, and a music program that is extremely diverse. For some of the students identified here as musos, their interest in music seemed part of their engagement with the school at a range of levels. Jake was a gifted musician, but he was also centrally involved in the sports program of the school. Ben and Aaron placed a great emphasis on music, but this was part of a broader range of activities, including some not organised formally by the school. Julian and Sebastian, on the other hand, centred music as a way of understanding the subcultures at the school. They described the music first and then the groups of students who listened to particular artists. For them, music was a way of making meaning. While Ben, Aaron, and Jake all nominated jazz as their music of interest, Sebastian and Julian had been punks and had forgone this strict identification in order to jump between groups. Similarly, instead of nominating one instrument as the others had, they played a 'small orchestra' between them. Unlike the others, Julian and Sebastian did not discuss any nonmusic extracurricula activities. At Leafy Suburbs College music was offered as part of the formal curriculum as well as being embedded in a range of optional activities. Most of these boys included music in their formal school curriculum and yet none of them nominated it as an area of study they wished to continue. Only two mentioned music as part of a career and then only as a context for engineering in the case of Aaron, and graphics in the case of Julian and Sebastian. Being a muso did not offer the income or the stability that these boys sought in their future lives. This will be discussed further in the chapter dealing with students' imagined futures.

The music program at the school was large and diverse. It included a range of options that included classical music and some jazz-inspired programs. Singing was well represented with soloists and ensembles performing. However, there was an absence of what might be termed popular music. Students who learned guitar did so outside the formal school curriculum and contributed to bands organised through the school but on an informal basis. For some, this was part of what made the school conservative and exclusive. One member of staff argued that there had been a ground swell over more recent years to shift this emphasis. Most notably this had been done through the organisation of a talent quest for students. Rather than part of the formal school program, this took the form of a series of lunchtime performances over a week. These performances highlighted popular music and in some instances included students who were not involved in the established school music program but who were serious musicians outside school. There was minimal staff involvement and commonly, staff involved were not music staff. Students were seen to own this activity and the performances expressed their musical preferences rather than those formalised through formal school structures. It was during this talent quest that students performed music such as rock, heavy metal, and punk. Some staff argued that there was resistance to this program, particularly by music staff. For these staff, the talent quest became transgressive. Music staff attitudes were read variously as resistance premised on fatigue or conservatism. For some, it was a matter of staff in the existing program, already overburdened and under-resourced, being understandably reluctant to take on more. For others, it was explained in almost conspiratorial terms. Music was a power base within the school, something that represented the core of a program that streamed students and privileged dominant forms of knowledge and learning. Replacing violins with electric guitars had great symbolic worth — it was a case of removing a foundational brick from the wall (with deference to Pink Floyd!)

It is possibly worthwhile to consider participation in the school music program. In the junior year levels, the majority of students were included in various ways. The year level bands involved most students, while the orchestra, various ensembles, and the variety of vocal groups seemed more exclusive. In senior year levels, the number of students involved in the program declined, which reflected the move away from a general curriculum to one increasingly premised on student subject preferences. While it was possible to continue in the band or orchestra and not continue music (instrumental and theory) as part of the formal curriculum, this was unusual given the increasing pressure on students as they approached senior year levels. To someone on the outside looking in, it did seem that the music program included the full range of students at the school. Nonetheless, some of the clichés about the type of students who do particular types of music were apparent. 'Asian' and 'Russian' students were extremely well represented in classical music. Openly gay and bisexual boys were involved in musical theatre. Singers and dancers were most often girls, particularly from the junior year levels. Percussionists were most often junior boys. And jazz luminaries were most often senior boys.

The concert had been rumoured for some time and eventually news of it became official through the school website. This was to be the first school jazz concert and there was much excitement, in part because former students were rumoured to be involved — most importantly, Harvey Armstrong. Harvey was a former student who had become an acclaimed performer both in Australia and overseas. His was a brand of fusion music that was underpinned by a jazz tradition learned at Leafy Suburbs College. Students bought tickets in advance and interest extended to those who previously had been at the school. This was different to the concerts attended by devoted parents and grandparents that dotted the school calendar at regular and predictable intervals. There was a very different ambience to this event.

The curtains parted and the first performance was by a group of professional jazz musicians, one of whom was on the staff. This teacher was performing with his peers — a way of bringing the real world into the school. At the conclusion of this four-song set, the stage was occupied by various acts. Most commonly these centred on current students, particularly those who would be sitting for their Year 12 exams in music performance in the forthcoming weeks — a self-assured male percussionist who moved seamlessly between several xylophones and various drum kits; a young man whose trumpet playing pierced the auditorium with cascades of sound that evoked much clapping and cheering from peers, parents, and staff, a Year 12; female clarinet player whose downcast gaze and awkward shuffle to centre-stage evoked sympathy; and a young woman in the back stalls, who was cheered through her first trumpet solo, despite this being her sixth year of playing the instrument at the school. Staff moved in and out of these performances, mostly in background roles as the need arose. However, most excitement was reserved for Mr Ryan who took responsibility for the senior jazz band and who was held in high regard both as a musician and a teacher. He had been at the school for many years and was associated with the success of the students who had become acclaimed musicians after leaving the school.

The senior jazz band was featured near the end of the program and Mr Ryan took the time to thank soloists by name. He specifically noted the contribution of three young women who were featured on piano, trumpet, and clarinet, respectively. 'Please put your hands together for Amy, Melanie, and Katrina. We are particularly proud of the girls in the jazz band' The highlight of the evening was Harvey and two other former students. All were in their early twenties and each was introduced in the context of the bands they were now part of and the venues at which they had regular 'gigs'. Harvey was the highlight and the epitome of good grace given the fuss that surrounded his inclusion in the program. He thanked Mr Ryan with the statement, 'If it wasn't for this man, none of us would be playing music now.' The climax of the evening was a performance by Harvey and Mr Ryan with the latter deferring to his former student in a gesture filled with humility (about his own playing) and pride (in his teaching).

A particular type of charismatic masculinity flooded the stage. It was premised on an understated self-assurance. There was a communion of shared interest, a pecking order, and an understanding of how to earn respect and move through the established ranks. The body language and the eye contact spoke volumes about the place of each player and the camaraderie between them. This unspoken way of being musical exemplified a type of 'men's secret society'. This is the type of society women experience as exclusive, describe to each other with enormous clarity and mutual recognition, and that men dismiss as a product of their imagination. The public acknowledgment of Melanie, Amy and Katrina consolidated their place outside this 'secret society'. Real members already knew their worth.

Chapter 10

Being Mercenary — The Politics of Performance

> On the level of the self, a fundamental component of day-to-day activity is *simply* that of choice. Obviously, no culture eliminates choice altogether in day-to-day affairs, and all traditions are effectively choices among an indefinite range of possible behaviour patterns. Yet, by definition, tradition or established habit orders life within relatively set channels. Modernity confronts the individual with a complex diversity of choices and, because it is non-foundational, at the same time offers little help as to which options should be selected. Various consequences tend to follow.
>
> (Giddens 1991:80, original emphasis)

Students interviewed for this study identified particular subcultures as existing within their school. They connected these subcultures with ways of dressing, specific types of music, and attitudes to school. Whilst these students described each other as being from particular subcultures, few accepted membership of a subculture. Instead, they reflected on how others might construct them as a 'muso' or a 'nerd', for example, and then described how such identifications were inappropriate. For some students, it was a case of reclaiming and redefining the categories. Others explained how they functioned at the crossroads of subcultures or moved between various ones. Whilst strategies altered, it was clear that none of these students wanted to be seen in straightforward ways as belonging. Instead, they upheld categories by naming them in order to disown them. In this chapter,

I wish to consider how student subcultures and the everyday experience of schooling might intersect. How do students who have been labelled 'nerds', for example, describe their teachers, the school curriculum, or the school's reputation? In order to explore such questions, I have to privilege the way students have been categorised by their peers, rather than the students' own self-identifications. While there are clear disadvantages in this way forward, given these students' reluctance to own a label, it seems the only means of considering differences between various groups.

Leafy Suburbs College has been characterised as a 'pretend private' school. It is a government school with a strict uniform code and a range of facilities, which whilst modest in comparison to elite independent and Catholic schools, are better than those offered by many government schools. Students are offered a wide range of extracurricula activities and achieve results that enable entry into elite universities. I have argued that as a government school, Leafy Suburbs College has relatively limited resources and has to make strict choices about the use of these resources. Within the logic of the market, if it is to brand itself as an academic school, it has to do more with less. As a government school niche marketing itself as academic, it can provide only those choices that best facilitate results that work in favour of university entry. This is both a burden and a privilege for students, staff, and parents. Attending Leafy Suburbs College means a better chance of accessing higher education, which is a high priority. On the other hand, once enrolled, students, regardless of their backgrounds and preferences, need to conform to a particular set of practices that are arguably rigid. Students are regulated through reference to the privilege of enrolment, an opaque system that channels students most likely to achieve into the school, counsels those least likely to achieve, out of the school, and uses high demand for places as a means of reinforcing its message. It is in this sense that Leafy Suburbs College 'orders life within relatively set channels' and 'at the same time offers little help as to which options should be selected' (Giddens 1991:80). In this and the next chapter, I explore how students identified with various subcultures experience their school at the level of the every day (Smith 1987) and consider how they respond to the ordering of their lives and select options between the set channels. In Chapter 12, this process is considered in relation to how these students imagine their futures.

Several clear themes emerged from descriptions of the school made by staff, parents, and students. The school's reputation was referred to and linked to the fact that demand for places could not be met. The school's 'good reputation' was defined in relation to results which were produced through rigorous discipline. This discipline was linked to work expectations, strict uniform code, and the intolerance of aberrant behaviours such as drug taking, alcohol consumption, and violence. In the case of some interviewees, most commonly staff, good results were also linked to a school community that took school seriously. Most students discussed teachers and teaching at length. This issue will be discussed separately in the following chapter. Whilst these students are associated with particular subcultures, they are not understood as representative of these subcultures.

- Every individual is important. We recognise and appreciate the diversity of our students and the enrichment it brings to our school environment.

- We nurture and support the growth of all individuals as they seek to achieve their personal, educational, moral and social goals, developing in each a sense of self-worth and self-respect.

- We enable students to reach their potential by providing a broad range of choice in curricular and extracurricular programs.
(Leafy Suburbs College Teaching and Learning Charter)

I wouldn't call them a supportive school ... they'll help you a lot, but if you need help they don't help you as much. (Daniel)

The teaching and learning charter for Leafy Suburbs College is unambiguous in expressing a range of beliefs and values about student identity. Individuals are important, diversity is important, and helping students achieve their goals and potential through diversified curricula is important. Nonetheless, students, including successful students, do not experience their school in this way. Daniel, an academically successful student, feels that the school supports those who need support least. Others involved in this study shared Daniel's sentiment. We need to understand this difference between intention and lived experience without vilifying the school and its teachers or eulogising youthful chagrin as the immediate response to recognising the gap between what is hoped for relative to what is. As adults, how do we explain and justify to young people our complicity in a range of practices that we simultaneously show disdain for and yet promulgate? In this case, the strategies that work, that get students over the line and into university are the same practices experienced as uncaring. It is such a tight and dangerous space between discomfort and success that is of interest. Do all students share Daniel's view or is it those from particular subcultures who experience their school as uncaring? Through the interviews, it became obvious that students' responses to these issues were not tied to their academic success in any straightforward way. In some ways, it was the students who were most adept with the pedagogies of performance, the high achievers, who were the most scathing about the way schooling was done at Leafy Suburbs College.

Each interview conducted with students, either in groups or individually, included a question asking them to describe what they thought were the positive aspects of their school. This was an attempt to deemphasise the negative. What follows draws on responses students made to this question.

The Everyday Experience According to Nerds

In Chapter 6, Stephen, Miread, Daniel, and Paul were introduced and described as 'nerds'. At the time of the interview, these students were in Year 10. The interview was conducted near the end of the school year when students at this level were being counselled by VCE coordinators. This is a rigorous process during which students are individually interviewed and on the basis of Year 10 results guided into Year 11 and 12 subjects. During this process, some students who are considered less well suited to the academic program offered at the school are advised to seek enrolment at neighbourhood schools with more flexible curricula. Commonly, students in this category, who leave Leafy Suburbs College, move to Alternative College, a relatively liberal government school. Uniform is not required there and students interviewed described it as caring and as adopting student-centred approaches. Alternative College was strong in the arts, including performing arts, and offered vocationally orientated subjects. The interview began thus:

GT: All right. Describe the things about the school that you think make it ... good basically.

Miread: Umm ...

Stephen: I'm not very happy with the school at the moment!

GT: You're not?

Stephen: No.

Daniel: The school is very ... efficient ... very, mercenary ...

Miread: Yeah ...

Daniel: It's very ... supportive of the people who do well.

Paul: Yeah, very supportive.

Miread: So, if you're achieving, you will achieve ...

Daniel: And they will help you 'til the end of the year.

Miread: But, yeah ...

Paul: If you don't show the dedication, they're not going to show you through.

Miread: So if you're that student, then it's good for you ... and yeah, so that's good. They push ...

GT: Ok, so if you're dedicated. Can you tell me, mercenary — what do you mean?

Paul: Yeah, Daniel, big word!

Daniel: Um, I mean, that they're very conscious about that sort of thing, and um ... the way they look at students I think, and the way they look at getting your money in and ... and as if money is more important than ... than anything really! Um ... I don't know what it's like in other schools because every school needs money and I realise that, but um ... I do think this school takes a particularly hard line on the getting your money in, and getting the fees in.

Stephen: Well, they do because one of the selection criterias for getting into Year 7 is um, past academic achievements and the ability to play a musical instrument, so obviously if you're a good academic you might win awards and stuff for the school which generates money for them.

Daniel: It generates prestige, more than money.

Stephen: That too ... which gives them, well, they can get grants from the government and stuff for being a good school.

Daniel: We do get grants for music especially.

Stephen: Exactly, so that's why ... that's one thing that they have.

Daniel: I wouldn't call them a supportive school, but I would call them a very ... they'll help you a lot, but if you need help, they don't help you as much.

Paul: That's the best way to put it.

Daniel: You kind of get the feeling that they're running a marks-generated thing ...

GT: A what?

Daniel: A marks-generated, something that generates good marks and good results at Year 12, rather than ...

Miread: Like we're not people, we are the scores above our heads ... like potential scores.

Stephen: Like 'You, you'll get 95, and you'll get 82, go away.'

Miread: Yeah, exactly.

Daniel: Like trying to run our school, they do it quite well. Look, and they get really great marks, I mean half our Year 12s last year got over 90.

GT: So does that impress you? Like do you see it as something that works and therefore you're happy to be part of?

Miread: Well, it depends.

Paul: As long as you're within that top 10%, but if you're below it, you're going to have to review your options of school.

Daniel: But, I think this is a brilliant school for academic achievers and shocking for people who aren't.

GT: You all agree on that?

Miread: Yeah. Because I'm leaving this year — I'm doing different subjects, that's why — but I think if I stayed at Leafy Suburbs College I'd definitely get a higher mark, but be not as happy with what I'm doing. That's what I sort of see because like, they would push me and sort of make me work harder, but I'd prefer to do things on my own, I'm just like that. I'd prefer to work at myself and do it my way. So people that don't really fit in the system, they get shuffled out of it.

GT: So were you shuffled out, or have you chosen to go?

Miread: I've chosen to go. They wanted me to stay because I've got good marks.

Stephen: Oh …

Miread: My brother went here as well, and he's gone to Alternative College as well, and he was getting bad marks, so he was asked to leave a few times. Because they didn't want to expel him … they didn't want to expel him and they said that — they're not allowed to expel him for nothing — but they said that 'We suggest you leave and would be better in the workforce because no other school will take you.' So, this is in Year 9, telling a Year 9 guy that he should you know … that school's not going to take him. It comes up to me and I've been getting straight A+'s and they're saying 'Oh, no you shouldn't leave, no, you're great!' And I'd say 'Oh, but I want to do these subjects' and they'd say 'No, do Maths, do Biology.'

GT: So the subjects you want to do they don't offer?

Paul: No.

GT: What are they?

Paul: They offer strict subjects, they're all academic science subjects.

Miread: I'm doing Politics, Philosophy, International Studies um, I'm doing Year 12 History and English …

GT: None of those are offered here?

Paul: Year 12 English is.

Miread: We have Year 12 International and …

Stephen: We have Politics, but it's dodgy … Politics was cancelled.

Miread: We all tried to do political studies, but they didn't let us; we didn't have enough people.

Daniel: Me and Miread had the same problem this year; Miread chose to leave and do better subjects and I chose to stay and do something that I wasn't quite happy with but will probably get better marks.

It is clear that these students understand the culture of success cultivated at the school and how this is linked to entry requirements, prestige, and resources. This recognition is not surprising as part of the school culture is inculcating in the students an understanding of the privilege of enrolment. Part of the established discourse, reiterated at school assemblies, for example, includes entry and exit numbers, so much so that junior students can tell you that as many, if not more, students were denied entry as those who were enrolled. As indicated by the interview, senior students can describe the VCE results for the school. This is the 'jewel in the crown' of the way the school represents itself — what makes it valuable and the raison d'être for everything else. The corollary of this is the understanding that if you don't perform academically, you are pressured to leave. This is illustrated through Miread's comment, that students are not people, but instead a potential score. These students also subscribe to a politics of subject selection — they describe subjects that are interesting and subjects that help you do well, and in their eyes, these are sometimes mutually exclusive choices. These four students understood the game of getting over the line, what was required, what were the benefits, and what was at stake. And each student responded differently to this realisation. Miread had decided to leave Leafy Suburbs College and go somewhere that offered more freedom, but also by her estimation, more risk. By attending Alternative College she believed she was reducing her chances of getting into university, she would have to work harder and be more self-reliant than if she stayed at Leafy Suburbs College. The others had all decided to stay at Leafy Suburbs College because of what it offered, including the extracurricula program.

Supporting Good Results

These students argued that the school was mercenary and focused not on them as people, but instead, in Miread's terms, on 'the potential score above their heads'. They argued that only the successful students were provided with support. This was not a view held by others. Jake, the charismatic pianist described in Chapter 8, experienced the school as caring and supportive. He had lower aspirations than Stephen, Miread, Paul, and Daniel, and represented himself as a student who needed to work harder to get better results. Yet he was most appreciative of the efforts of his teachers.

> GT: Can you describe the things about the school that you appreciate the most?
>
> Jake: Well, I guess, what's good about this school is the teachers are all willing to give up a lot of their time to see you succeed. Like I went to Miss Campari and she had a couple of classes on and she got another teacher in just so she could work with us before our exams. And it's just things like that, and

they're willing to give up after-school hours and just to really help you out, which I think is one of the key things. And also they push you to strive for your best. It's not like, 'Oh yeah, if you do it, you do it'. They sort of get you to do it. Well, it's sort of bad at the time because you're like 'Bloody teachers, I hate them!' but at the end of the day you're going to look back and think, if I hadn't had that I might not have done so well.

GT: 'They sort of get you to do it', can you explain that a bit more?

Jake: Well, they make sure you get the deadlines in on time, otherwise you have consequences. And if you do have troubles at home, they'll give you allowances and say, 'All right, you can hand it in by this date', and they talk to you and stuff. So it's a really good relationship at this school between students and teachers, I think.

Unlike Daniel and his friends who described the school as mercenary, Jake described a school culture that cultivated success through instilling in students the discipline of working to deadlines, being well organised, and conscientious. He experienced the school as flexible and accommodating of students' personal problems. It was also a school where teachers gave their time generously and in response to students' needs. There are many issues that could explain such stark differences in perception. A major factor relates to year-level. At the time of the interview, Jake was in the final weeks of Year 11. As students progressed through the school, their experience of the school altered, something many of them commented upon. Teachers treated senior students differently, they were afforded more privileges, the pressures of the VCE were understood, and every effort was made to support them through the final stages of their school and to achieve the best possible results.

This approach was particularly evident through the persona of Ms Fotiadis. As the Vice Principal for the Senior School, she had responsibility for VCE. She was tireless and student focused. Students saw her as someone who championed their cause, including with other teachers with whom they may have poor relations. Students looked forward to being under her charge. One parent stated that 'If it wasn't for Ms Fotiadis, my son would never have finished school'. He described her as accommodating of his son's lack of focus. She was flexible and understanding, choosing caring approaches and negotiating differences rather than standing by formalities and exercising power in strident ways and to prove a point. Yet she was known to be 'no nonsense'. She could be very hard hitting, making clear what was expected. If she knew students were serious about trying, almost everything was possible; if they weren't serious, they were left in no doubt about expectations and consequences. She had the respect of her colleagues and this made negotiating differences between students, teachers, and parents successful. In many ways, she epitomised the wholesome version of the school, that anything was possible if you tried hard enough. Jake had accepted this without looking behind this as the official rendition of schooling. Miread and her friends, while finding it easier than Jake to perform at a high standard, articulated their cynicism about the official storyline.

Standard Measures

Sophia, Anna, and Lucy were described by students as 'wogs' and introduced in Chapter 7. Sophia was of Greek extraction and Anna's mother was Maltese. Lucy had come to Leafy Suburbs College from a single-sex Catholic school and was leaving to attend Alternative College, the less traditional neighbouring government school. She was part of the 'wog' group, but did not indicate having an ethnic minority background. These girls did not have high aspirations. They were not involved in any of the extracurricula programs at Leafy Suburbs College. Relative to other interviewees, they appeared disengaged. Their attitudes to the school reinforced my sense of their disengagement. When asked what they liked about the school, Sophia began with the following comment:

Sophia: They like to keep you on track with your work, like, don't want you to miss anything and they always want you to hand things in and stuff. It's annoying sometimes because you always have to be on track, but it's good in a way, because they really want you to try — they want you to do well in that subject.

Anna: Whereas sometimes other schools I hear about they're not ... it doesn't get to them as much that people are falling behind because it's their own choice, whereas Leafy Suburbs College's on your back forcing you to do your best — well not forcing you but encouraging you.

GT: And is that a good thing?

Anna: Yeah, it is a good thing, in the long run, I guess. At this stage, it's our decision if we ... it's up to us — but yeah, it is good for our education.

GT: What don't you like about it?

Sophia: It's a bit strict on uniform! Some of the teachers are a bit ... I think they take their job way too seriously.

GT: Can you talk about that?

Sophia: Um ... I don't know how to say it .... Some teachers are really uptight about work, if it's not up to their standards, it's not good enough, but it might be up to your standards, so they'll give you a lower mark if it's not up to their standard but it's your best standard.

Anna: It's harder when the teachers are different because some of the more younger teachers are more relaxed and laid back and you can get along with them, and you enjoy going to class. Some of the others you don't get along well with, you don't have a good friendship with them, and sometimes you can hand something into them and it might be a C+ standard and another teacher might see it and think it's a B+. It's just different with different teachers and different classes.

Anna and Sophia capture the contradiction of being at school that is good for you because it makes you try hard, keeps you on track, and expects you to achieve and, in so doing, places a great deal of pressure on you. Despite trying, Sophia's best efforts do not meet the high standards expected of her by teachers. Her comment that her highest standard is not good enough hints at not coping well. Anna explained her relative lack of achievement differently. The difference between a C and B grade reflected differences between teachers and subjects. Despite the school being 'on your back forcing you to do your best', A grades did not come into the picture for these girls.

Performing Disengagement

Nadine and Amy, introduced in Chapter 7, were students who were described as 'blonde' or 'popular' girls. Their self-representation included camouflaging elements that could be misconstrued as 'nerdy'. They wanted to be seen as too busy socialising to do homework. Yet Nadine had high aspirations and had selected academic subjects for Year 11. She had chosen to do two types of mathematics, chemistry, physics, and a Year 12 subject as part of an accelerated program. Amy's program was less ambitious. Nadine described how her teachers had warned her that with her selection of subjects, she would have to work hard. This was something she described as 'stressful'. Nadine's comments about the school reflected what, in my mind, reiterated itself as feigned cynicism — part of her performing the 'blonde' schoolgirl.

GT:	Describe the things you most appreciate about the school.
Nadine:	Oh, well they're going to get us money by having an education.
Amy:	A good job, a good education.
Nadine:	It's like a good school, it's got a pretty good reputation as well.
Amy:	Teachers treat you good as well.
GT:	Why do you think the school's got a good reputation?
Nadine:	Um, I dunno.
Amy:	They push hard on us to do well.
Nadine:	Yeah, the people here that actually want to learn, they actually want to get an education and that sort of influences other people around them for them to want to do good. Whereas at some other schools people just don't care, and because they don't, that influences on everyone.

Nadine: I don't know! I think they got that before we were here. We have a pretty strict uniform and they're pretty strict compared to other schools, and there's not many druggies compared to other schools. So you don't really see many people with slicked-back blonde hair with black regrowth and eye makeup everywhere. If you see someone like that you'd think 'Oh, what school do they go to?'

Here, Nadine provides a reference to herself as bad for the school's reputation. This description remains unconvincing. In the next breath she describes the type of students who give schools a bad reputation. These are students who take drugs. She also describes such students with reference to their makeup and hair colour. The comment about 'black regrowth' paints a vivid picture. By contrast, Nadine and Amy present as wellgroomed, neat, and tidy and relative to some other girls, quite demure in their hairstyles and use of makeup. It is interesting to note their comment about strict uniform. It is something they value about their school in contrast to Anna, Sophia, and Lucy who agree that the uniform code is too strict and something their teachers take 'too seriously'. Nonetheless, Nadine and Amy believe that it is the results that distinguish their school.

GT: How do you think the school compares with others?

Nadine: I think it's pretty good … But yeah, compared to the private schools in the area the facilities aren't as good as like, some of them, but overall, the results we get are probably a lot better than the other public schools in the area.

Managing Performance

Ben and Aaron were two of the students identified as musos in Chapter 8. While dedicated to music, these boys had ambitions to enter law and engineering. They were involved with the Jewish community and Ben had immigrated to Australia from South Africa. They were very positive about Leafy Suburbs College and the opportunities it offered. They were interviewed at the end of Year 11.

GT: What do you appreciate about this school?

Aaron: I like how you can always get help from teachers, especially this year, like Year 7–10 are alright but Year 11 and 12 the teachers are really good and they're always available to help you and everything like that, so yeah, anytime you want help, I mean if you muck around in class they won't help you, but if you actually like pay attention in class and that, they'll help you whenever you want.

Ben: I also find that — definitely Year 11 and 12 the student/teacher relationship is more on a personal level not really just student/teacher. You can often talk to them when you've got a — like if you need help and stuff and yeah, they're very helpful when it comes to work, especially with Year 12 subjects

	they always give priority obviously to Year 12 students, which is probably a good thing. Yeah, also the high standard of like the work and stuff — I think Leafy Suburbs College is a good school as far as government schools go, they're one of the better ones. High standard of ethos.
GT:	Do you agree with that?
Aaron:	Yes, yes. Last year over two-thirds of people — over 50% of people got above 90 at the end, so I think it's a pretty successful school and plus the music program is probably better than a lot of other schools. Like all the little sound studios have got gear and everything like that. It's pretty good.
GT:	How do you think the school compares with others?
Ben:	I think in terms of the kids it produces like, you often find a lot of kids they're like better kids compared to — they don't have as many social problems I suppose with smoking and stuff, I find in our year-level, there's probably a minority that smoke compared to some other schools where probably a majority in Year 11 smoke, and just yeah, probably alcohol and drugs and stuff like that I find. I don't know they're kind of like proactive in sports and other things.
Ben:	Yes, I guess — well I went to King David primary school that's a private school and I don't know, my brother and sister both found that better than here, but I think this is a lot better because there they have really small classes and they're really focusing on you. When you get to uni that all just disappears, so this sort of prepares you more for university, I reckon, public school and that.
GT:	And you chose not to go there?
Ben:	My parents wanted me to go here and I also chose to go because I heard about the music program and that and I wanted to do better in my music and that.
GT:	What type of students do you think have succeeded?
Ben:	I'm just trying to think because I suppose like actually their school work or probably get the most out of school.
GT:	Well, you can talk about either.
Ben:	Well, I think if you want to get the most out of school, you can't just be a complete study freak all the time. You have to have a bit of a social life and obviously school is like — one of the main aspects of it is I suppose to make new friends and stuff — I mean when you're going to school.
Aaron:	Yeah, you have to work hard, but yeah, you also have to go out sometimes. My brother said, he didn't go out at all during his VCE year and he said it was the worst mistake he's ever made. He said you know, it got really monotonous and you really, like if you've got somewhere to be then you look forward to studying because you know at the end of it you know you're going out and stuff, so you've got to still work out as well.

GT: Did he do well?

Aaron: Yes, he did pretty well. He mucked up his English exam which he didn't do too well, but apart from that yes, and he still got a pretty high ENTER score, so he didn't do too bad, but he said he could have done much better if he went out a bit. He just stayed home the whole time.

Ben: I suppose probably students with a goal, if you know what you want to do or if you've got something that you want to achieve, I suppose you can work towards it and stuff because otherwise you just I suppose — like you don't have much, not much incentive to do any work and stuff. Got bored.

GT: And there are lot of kids like that here?

Ben: With like the people who want to achieve and that?

GT: Yes.

Ben: Yes, I'd say probably a lot of kids, yes. I'd say probably half in our year-level at least. At soon as it hits the end of Year 10/11, a lot of the students — there's a big change compared to — in their attitude towards the work, because they kind of think 'Oh yeah, I'm going to have to get somewhere after school'. It's just not going to be my life, so they kind of change and want to do well to get to where they want to go.

These two boys presented a very no-nonsense approach to their school. Leafy Suburbs College had what was described as a 'high standard of ethos' and this was evidenced by the types of students who attended the school. These were not the types who smoked, drank alcohol, and did drugs. Instead, the students at the school had high aspirations, were dedicated students, and achieved excellent results. But for these boys, school was also about the social networks, the opportunities to do other things, including music, and to learn independence. In this context, Aaron argues that his siblings who attended a private Jewish school, were mollycoddled, which in his estimation would disadvantage them when they entered university. There is an assumption here that school is about getting to university; what alters is the path taken to achieve this end. Ben and Aaron confirm Jake's experience of the teachers. During Years 11 and 12, there is no doubt in their minds as to the investment of time and effort made by teachers toward students' success. They do qualify this statement with the comment that 'I mean if you muck around in class, they won't help you, but if you actually like pay attention in class and that, they'll help you whenever you want'. This attitude lies some way between the extremely positive view Jake provides and the view expressed by Paul, Daniel, Miread, and Stephen that teachers only care about the students who need the least support. Again, it is worth noting that such a shift in emphasis may reflect the difference between being in Year 10 or Year 11. Paul and the others were commenting as Year 10 students who were being counselled about their final years of schooling. The others were presenting perspectives from within their final years of schooling. Finally, Ben and Aaron speak from within the group of students they identify as wishing to succeed. From this vantage point they identify a school ethos that they argue is critical if they are to achieve their aspirations.

Performing Below Par

Sebastian and Julian were described in detail in Chapter 9. They were interviewed at the end of the final exams when they were in the process of making university course selections. These students were intent on entering courses tangentially related to music, despite the central role of music in their lives. They had used music to frame their description of school subcultures and youth cultures more broadly. They described their friends as 'bare-footed bohemians' and presented as eclectic and avant-garde in their dress and manner. They were extremely thoughtful, sophisticated in their analysis, and produced a range of insights that hinted at deconstructive method learned through English Literature, a subject they held in high regard. Their responses to their school were particularly interesting. While they sported extreme hairstyles and valued clothing that made a statement, they nonetheless supported a range of practices at the school, including compulsory uniform that seemed ill matched to their general demeanour. However, it is worth noting in this context that these young men took pride in unsettling preconceptions and at various points within the interview I found it difficult to distinguish irony from straightforward description.

GT: Ok, describe the things you appreciate about this school.

Sebastian: Um, the music program is very good and there's so many opportunities. There's various bands to cater for pretty much everyone. There is no actual guitar teacher which I think is good because there are so many people who would want to be guitarists that they would have to hire more teachers than they were able to handle, but still, there is lots of good music out there, the band is great fun and there are so many things you can do through that. The environment is good.

GT: What would you change if you were the principal?

Sebastian: I would probably have some sort of gestapo thing policing the littering because that really does get on my nerves. The huge amounts of rubbish, garbage that seems to be generated. I wouldn't mind more grass. That would be about the only thing.

GT: More grass and less litter.

Julian: Yes.

Sebastian: I don't know, less litter, making students stop littering is actually fairly hard because we're generally lazy, can't be bothered walking that extra two metres to a bin.

GT: Kids could pick up their own litter.

Sebastian: True, in theory anyway, but normally you end up with a couple of students picking up everybody's litter.

These students' immediate response is to consider the school in relation to music and environmental issues. The use of 'gestapo' in this context is interesting, given its juxtaposition with littering and more grass, concerns often identified with the countercultural.

GT: How do you think this school compares to others?

Sebastian: No one in the company of their friends will admit to liking their own school, but I think that if anyone didn't want to be here, they wouldn't, like people I've known who've transferred to Alternative College, and all these other schools, and I think our school is actually really good. It's got a good balance of things. You know it's lacking in some areas, no drama department, but very few schools actually have a decent drama department. Most of them are run by English teachers which … certainly have the qualifications but. But I think they're putting the funding to good use. They're developing it really well. They've got up-to-date technology courses, computer labs and all that stuff, the teachers know their stuff and we get very adequate education. You hear stories about places like Alternative College being schools for dropouts and all that, and Leafy Suburbs College has a very good reputation, nothing like that sort of stuff. I think it's one of the better schools around.

School Ethos

Julian and Sebastian regularly refer to Alternative College in their exploration of Leafy Suburbs College. This is not uncommon. This neighbourhood government school stood in stark contrast to Leafy Suburbs College. Instead of uniform, strict discipline, and academic subjects, this school offered a flexible curriculum which emphasised the arts, no uniform, and an environment that allowed students to work at their own pace. The VCE results for this school were significantly lower than those for Leafy Suburbs College. It was common for students who left Leafy Suburbs College to go to Alternative College — to choose something completely different.

GT: Why do kids you know move to other schools?

Sebastian: Most of the ones we know have been having a problem with teachers and authority in general. One of our friends who went to Alternative College was having real trouble with just the way things were run, having uniform

	troubles, difficulty with teachers, just like the lack of freedom they were given in the kind of subjects they were doing, because at places like Alternative College it's a lot more ... more looser — a lot more free, and at the same time there's a lot more kind of specific courses, like rather than, instead of just having a straight music, perform all music styles, they've got courses to go into sound engineering and stage work and ...
Julian:	There's a lot more humanities-oriented subjects as well.
GT:	So are they happy there?
Sebastian:	Yes, from what I know, they are happy there.
Julian:	Yes, they're enjoying themselves immensely by all accounts.
Sebastian:	Although we did know one girl who went to Alternative College and was very ...
Julian:	Went for a couple of weeks then just went back to her old school, because it wasn't structured. That freedom is good but unfortunately it can lead to — if you can't cope with it — very unpleasant working conditions.
Sebastian:	Because with no one kind of on your back all the time it does tend to — you tend to not get anything done which has happened to me a couple of times in some classes, just in Art and stuff. Without that kind of constant regimented course structure, we kind of drift off, start to not do anything, lose focus.

Here we have a familiar theme. Leafy Suburbs College offers students the structure and discipline that allows them to work to their optimum ability. This is contrasted to Alternative College where students are allowed more freedom, including the freedom to do less work.

GT:	So you've not been tempted to go elsewhere?
Sebastian:	No, not really. Besides, we've got too many friends here that we kind of — it wouldn't really be worth at the later stage where we would have been aware enough to think about such things. It wouldn't have been worth the pain of you know, uprooting and making new friends and all of that, so I mean we would have only been actually thinking from about Year 10 or 11, so by that stage, we were kind of settled in too much.
Julian:	Yes, that's only when that sort of stuff started to matter and you started to become aware of all the choices that we could make. By that stage, we were quite at home here.
GT:	But to look at you — I don't want to be rude, but you don't look straight do you. I mean you know dreadlocks and all that, and that's obviously not been an issue here.
Sebastian:	But the school is willing to permit certain things although they have clamped down on dreadlocks now, which is lucky because we just happened to be out of here.

GT: Oh, so they're 'illegal' now?

Sebastian: Yes, they've suddenly become — they've brought it that little bit further in. They've kind of made it that little bit stricter which I think is good. I like the uniform at school because you know it helps the attitude you know, for all the arguments about losing individuality and style stuff, it's actually good, it helps maintain focus and all that sort of stuff.

Julian: Because you know with the uniform on you know you're going to school, you're kind of ...

Sebastian: You're not supposed to be at school to look good. I suppose if you're not comfortable with it, you kind of just work with it until the stage where you can escape it or ... go to a school without a uniform like Alternative College.

GT: Oh, they don't have uniforms there.

Sebastian: No, no.

Julian: The only requirement is shoes and shirt.

Sebastian: Yes, you have to wear shoes and you have to wear a shirt. Because they had a bit of a stage where everyone was turning up without wearing shoes and shirts because they kind of took advantage of the lack of uniform rules. It was quite a craze for a couple months.

In this sequence, Julian and Sebastian hit on issues that remain central to the concerns under consideration here. By the time students are old enough to understand what is going on and the alternatives, it's too late to make choices. The cost of changing schools in your senior years is enormous. Similarly, these boys make the point that while there is a strict uniform code, there is also flexibility — well at least for some students. The school made an effort to accommodate students worth accommodating — students who were academically competent, worked well in class, and immersed themselves in extracurricula activities. While extreme hairstyles were fine for Sebastian and Julian, for other students, the slightest move in that direction became a cause for harassment. These boys are happy with a uniform code flexible enough to accommodate their priorities. School is not synonymous with looking good. It is a matter of conforming until you can 'escape' and if you find this too difficult you need to change schools.

GT: Ok, so in what type of things do you think you'll succeed?

Julian: Oh, that's a hard one. Succeed in what ways? Balance ...

Sebastian: Probably to succeed academically, they need to be fairly motivated and kind of driven. They kind of need to ...

GT: Hold on one person said balance and one person said driven.

Julian: Balanced.

Sebastian: Well, you go first — balanced.

Julian: Balance between social and academic, so you don't do too much of either because the kids who go way into academic either focus themselves too much and become unable to deal with other things or burn out and be unable to work. That almost happened with us.

Sebastian: A couple of years back we kind of — before we got into VCE we were kind of very conscientious little buggers, and yes …

Julian: All of a sudden we just started becoming really slack and we …

Sebastian: And we kind of — it's only like at the beginning of Year 11 I kind of looked back and realised how much I was not enjoying myself, how difficult it had all been.

Julian: We didn't really notice any of that sort of stuff until about halfway through last year.

Sebastian: We only kind of thought you know and looked back on how difficult we'd made everything for ourselves, so yeah …

Julian: Not making it difficult for yourself because in some ways it's easier because you know you don't have teachers on your back threatening to expel, suspend, fail you, all that sort of stuff.

Sebastian: Which although we are studying and relaxed, we still haven't had any problems with that. We don't get into any trouble at school or anything like that, so we've managed to kind of juggle, fairly, very good marks, with — there goes modesty — good marks with a kind of more relaxed attitude, so we're not kind of stressing or burning ourselves out or anything like that.

Julian: It would be just the balance — just the balance between relaxation and application, just you know be able to work hard but also be able to let off steam.

Sebastian: I think at — for school academics and stuff, you do need to be much more driven and focused. You need to kind of — if you're able to get behind yourself when there's nobody else you know to be on your back about it.

Julian: That's what — um where we used to fall down with, motivating ourselves. You have to be quite self-motivated if you're going to do all the extra study and homework and revision that academic excellence requires.

GT: But aren't you academically inclined?

Sebastian: Oh, we're pretty good. We're not …

Julian: We're academically excellent if we push ourselves and work at it, but otherwise you can descend into mediocrity basically …

Sebastian: Yeah, I mean we're not dux material, but we're kind of the "A" students.

GT:	Well, who does better than 'A'?
Julian:	Because all 'A+'; no deviation from the straight 'A+', straight 'A' like we're not too distraught we get 'B's' or the odd 'C'.
Sebastian:	Occasionally — it's not a really important thing for us, so yeah … maybe it's just priorities.
Julian:	Yes, although success is a difficult thing to try to define.
Sebastian:	Because you can have academic success, monetary success.
Julian:	You know you could live without a job and if you're enjoying it, then you'll be successful, you know if that's all you wanted and that's successful.

Sebastian and Julian establish a dialogue here in which they mediate each other's responses and come to a middle point on which there is agreement. Success is about balance. It is also about drive. Eventually, they compromise their positions to agree that success is about balance and drive, the drive to be balanced. They are academically competent and see themselves as capable of achieving A+ grades. But such results earmark 'dux material', a status to which they do not aspire. A+ students have lost balance, have become fixated on achieving results. Instead, they believe students should not 'burn themselves out' striving. Students need to be motivated, need teachers to provide structure and discipline in order to remain so, but also need to balance application and relaxation. By doing enough to get good marks, Julian and Sebastian also avoid the pressures that come from not doing what is expected of them. They do not wish to deal with the pressures linked to underperformance either. By avoiding A+ and getting A and B grades instead, they are able to remain relaxed. Remaining relaxed, in this context, intimated the ultimate muso persona. Yet relaxed achievement was not possible for all students; indeed, some strived and achieved poorly nonetheless. Such students did not seem to enter Julian and Sebastian's frame of reference.

Disciplining Performance

- All individuals are to be valued and treated with respect.
- Students can expect to learn in a secure environment without disruption or intimidation.
- Students have an obligation to care for and maintain a clean and hygienic environment.
- Teachers have a right to expect that they well be able to teach in an orderly and cooperative environment.
- Parents have a right to expect that their children will be educated in a secure environment in which care, courtesy, and respect for the rights of others are encouraged.

- Parents have an obligation to support the school in its effort to maintain a positive teaching and learning environment.

- Principals and staff have an obligation to fairly, reasonably and consistently implement the Student Code of Conduct.

- All members of the College community should strive to eliminate discrimination based on race, religion, gender or physical impairment.

(Leafy Suburbs College Student Code of Conduct)

Most students had left the school at least half an hour ago. In a room adjacent to the general office and the Principal's room sat a group of mainly male students. The atmosphere was sombre and the discomfort was palpable. There were no smiles, just the shuffling of restless feet that seemed too big for the bodies of the young men who owned them. The bespectacled teacher sitting at the front desk looked downward and the expression on her experienced face implied resignation rather than commitment to the task at hand. This was the day's detention class and it was not unusual for the same faces to reappear.

There is another story behind a school culture, which pressures students to perform. It may not suit all learners, including those who may prove to be good academic 'investments'. At the time of the interview Dimitri was in Year 9. Like many adolescent boys, he seemed uncomfortable in a body that had grown too rapidly. He was taller than many of his teachers, broad shouldered, with lots of dark hair and the blemishes that characterise those his age. He had a quiet charm that occasionally peeked through a type of broodiness. He answered questions with an economy of words that nonetheless expressed careful thinking. He wore his uniform with no telltale signs of belonging to any particular subculture. Many expected him to identify as a 'wog' because his appearance reflected a southern European heritage. In fact, he stated that his mother was Greek but not his father. Despite this, Dimitri had no affiliation with the 'wogs' who he described as 'gangster types' in a similar way to Sebastian and Julian. These were students who 'kind of act like a stereotypical male adolescents that you'd expect to see in a FuBu [brand name] jacket prowling the streets at night'. Dimitri did not think that these students were as tough as they made out to be. He described how some of these boys in his year-level had made fun of him after he declined their invitation to join their group.

In general terms, Dimitri was happy at the school, but argued that some of the teachers and their teaching methods needed to be reviewed by the Principal. This comment possibly reflected the problems he was having at the school. In his previous year of schooling, Dimitri had been in constant trouble with a number of his teachers and, as a result, with his year-level coordinators. He was rarely rude, often talkative, distracted, and distracting of others. He did not work in class, did not work at home, and failed to meet basic work requirements. As a result, his grades were very poor. Yet he was polite, inquisitive, and described as extremely capable by staff on the basis of his contributions to class discussion or test results. In Years 7 and 8, he had failed to make friends, had not got involved in any extracurricula activities, and had experienced some bullying. He was understood to be different, as not fitting in and somewhat enigmatic. Dimitri commented as follows when asked about the type of student who did well at the school:

Dimitri: It varies I think um you can't really say one personality type um does well. They have the kind of people who are quiet achievers and then you have other people who are loud and popular and they can also be good achievers. The only the way you can really tell is being in their class. Generally, the nerds do really well; the quiet achievers, they're the ones who get the extreme marks.

GT: You've been in trouble with teachers — would you like to talk about that?

Dimitri: Um I don't mind. Anything in particular.

GT: Describe what happened?

Dimitri: Um from what I know the teachers I had last year complained about my lack of work in class and my loudness in class. And the coordinators, my year-level coordinators, um decided to put me on an organisation card. This is basically something you must bring to every class and get the teacher to sign, that you have all your books and equipment and have written in your homework. The only thing this achieved with me was a lot of detentions and one in-school suspension.

GT: So this didn't change your attitude to work?

Dimitri: Not really. I found the only change it did was negative. It wasted a lot of my time, not only through detention but my constant presence at the coordinators' office. I think this year I've changed on my own accord and I don't think it was because of any teacher pushing me into it or trying to.

GT: So what changed your attitude?

Dimitri: Um I'm not entirely sure; I may have just matured with my academic attitude. Or maybe I just felt a bit better being more free; maybe that helped it.

GT: Do you think the school was trying to get rid of you?

Dimitri: Yes, it certainly felt that way near the end of last year, and this year I was put into a class away from my class and before the semester started I was moved again. When I tried to get out of this classroom because I knew I wasn't going to get along well with anyone in the class, my coordinators both last year and this year, ignored me. I think this may have been a result from my reputation in Year 8.

GT:	Why did you know you wouldn't get along with the kids in that class?
Dimitri:	I'd already spent two years with those people in my year-levels and you get to know other people in your level through sport and music, not to mention hearing about them from other people or seeing them at lunchtime.

Dimitri described a tight and relentless process of surveillance that had been imposed on him by his year-level coordinators. Each classroom teacher had to comment on his behaviour and he had to report to coordinators at the beginning and end of each day. His parents were also expected to sign the card. Any adverse comment by any teacher led to an after-school detention. These would cumulate into an in-house suspension and in turn an external suspension whereby the student had to stay home. These were taken seriously and details of such matters were kept on student files and could be used to support a case for expulsion in the future. This procedure and its possible consequences were well known to students. Dimitri had been given many detentions and an in-house suspension. Eventually, he had been given a three-day external suspension that he described as trivial.

GT:	Three-day suspension isn't trivial. What did the teachers think you had done wrong?
Dimitri:	Um I don't remember too much about it, but from my memory it was an accumulative thing to do with my organisation card.
GT:	So you weren't working in class enough?
Dimitri:	Um I can't really remember to be honest. I was um watched closely by the coordinators last year and through my lack of um classwork or homework they decided to send me to the school psych [school counsellor] um she thought I should be tested to see whether it was my intelligence level or whether it was some other reason. The result of this test showed that I was quite well above-average in almost all of the factors especially reading, when English was meant to be one of my weaker subjects.
GT:	So how did you feel about this?
Dimitri:	Um I wasn't really sure how to feel. I'd always been told to get up and do it. To be honest I don't really understand what was going on. I wasn't sure why I wasn't doing the work.
GT:	What did the coordinators think of the above-average test results?
Dimitri:	I can't remember ever talking to them about the subject. The coordinators basically told me that they would rather have someone else in my spot who did work and as we are told very often at our school there are hundreds of people lining up to get in because of the good reputation, which to be honest, almost everyone gets sick of.

Dimitri had been performing well below his potential. In his first two years of schooling at Leafy Suburbs College, he had been disengaged and had not met the school expectations regarding behaviour and work requirements. The school response to his disengagement was aggressive management through a system of surveillance that he describes as wasting his time and therefore compounding rather than solving the problem. He does not know why he did not conform to expectations of him, yet does not imply that the expectations were unreasonable in any way. Feeling pushed out of the school had not made the difference, neither had being in a class without friends. Instead, he offers maturing as the reason for his change in attitude. He cannot remember how the coordinators responded to his positive test results, but does remember their comment that he was occupying a place at the school that others wanted — a comment he described as something 'almost everyone gets sick of'.

Students like Dimitri brought out differences in teaching philosophy. While his particular coordinators took the approach they did, other coordinators argued that once Dimitri had been targeted, the surveillance became relentless and in this context, it was difficult for a student like him not to accumulate crosses against their name. As a government school, Leafy Suburbs College needed to make a case to the regional office before a student could be asked to leave. The necessary 'evidence' could be accumulated with enough effort. For some students, staying at Leafy Suburbs College in itself requires hard work. Over recent years there has been increasing pressure on the school to curtail selective enrolment. Nonetheless, getting into the school is half the battle of staying. Some students are made to feel more welcome than others, a process that requires being able to read into the future. One staff member explained:

> You can picture the kids that come in Year 7 that they're going to be one of the exit ones. Um ... aren't particularly academic and don't particularly want to try, and don't have a habit, or don't perhaps have expectations from family, that they will put in the discipline that's needed. I would guess there are probably about twenty kids who would leave the school at about Year 10 or 11 looking for an alternative to what we offer.

Giddens (1991) reminds us that a fundamental component of day-to-day activity relates to choice on the level of the self. In the context of a school such as Leafy Suburbs College, students are given harsh lessons in choice making with little guidance and the possibility of weighty consequences. For students like Sebastian and Julian, the choice to work below par still means getting A grades. For Sophia, on the other hand, the choice is whether or not to keep working diligently when her grades hover between C and B. Lucy has made a choice to leave her second secondary school in order to attend Alternative College. Dimitri has made a choice to stay at Leafy Suburbs College despite negative experiences at the school. He chooses to conform not because of teacher surveillance but in spite of it, a choice he attributes to his increasing maturity. As the staff member quoted above notes, kids leave 'looking for an alternative to what we offer'. This sentiment is echoed in Sebastian's comment that 'if you're not comfortable with it, you kind of just work with it until the stage where you can escape it or go…'. While it is important to note that this may not be a school philosophy premised on student centeredness, the argument being framed here is that this has a lot to do with marketisation. A government school does not have the resources to be all things to all students. As an academic school, Leafy Suburbs College has to do more with less and this leads to some fairly heavy-handed choices. Perhaps such choices are the price that has to be paid in order for students from public schools to enter elite universities. Clearly not all choices are equal and not all choices are equally available. In Chapter 11, I wish to consider this aspect of choosing in relation to students imagined futures and how students associated with various subcultures mediate choices about identity in relation to schooling and its outcomes. However, before doing this, I will consider school discipline in more detail in the following chapter.

Chapter 11

Disciplining for Reputation

Student Rights
All student at Leafy Suburbs College have the right to:

- feel safe and be safe.
- be treated with courtesy and respect.
- learn without interference.
- work and play without discrimination or harassment.
- voice their opinions in an appropriate manner.
- participate in decision-making in appropriate forums.

Student Responsibilities
Students at Leafy Suburbs College are expected to:

- take advantage of the opportunities provided by the college.
- treat their peers, teachers and members of the community with courtesy and respect.
- respect the right of other students to learn.
- use appropriate manners toward teachers and respect their right to teach.

- respect school property and maintain a clean environment.
- respect the property of others.
- behave in a manner which brings credit to the College.
- behave in a manner which does not include discrimination or harassment.
- fulfil obligations with respect to communications between the college and home.
- respect common law and community values.
- use acceptable language at all times.

(Leafy Suburbs College Code of Conduct)

Leafy Suburbs College has a reputation for academic excellence and good discipline. The type of school uniform and the way its wearing is policed becomes one of the markers for a 'serious' school. At the school, boys are expected to wear a tie at all times, including while travelling to and away from school. The exception to this is when the temperature reaches 35 degrees Celsius and special permission is given for top shirt buttons to be undone and ties removed. Shirts must be tucked in at all times. Girls are disciplined for wearing makeup and boys and girls know that 'extreme' hairstyles and jewellery are not tolerated. While such uniform codes are common at most independent and Catholic schools, within the government sector there is a wide range of difference. At one extreme, there are schools such as Leafy Suburbs College where there is insistence on strict uniform and related discipline codes, while at the other extreme there are schools with no uniform. In between, there are schools that adopt a minimalist uniform policy, such as the wearing of an inexpensive windcheater displaying the school logo with pants of a particular colour. Students at Leafy Suburbs College responded to their school's uniform policy in various ways. There were some students who understood it as a positive aspect of their school and one that contributed to its good reputation. Others considered both the type of uniform and the harsh discipline needed to ensure it was worn arcane. Two boys explained:

Paul: Ties! Ties are so stupid! They were created as a dish rag back in like the sixteenth century! They're not needed, they make you ...

Daniel: That's where you get the noose thing ...

Paul: Ties, I'd get rid of ties ...

The school uniform, for many students, became a symbol of the authority teachers exercised over them. Many of the students involved in the study were not against uniform per se but felt that at their school policing of uniform was unreasonably strict. Jake was happy with the school and was most positive about the teachers and what the school offered more generally. Yet on the issue of uniform, he made the following comment:

> I guess I'd change the policy on uniform. I think they're a bit harsh on it ... they're sort of ... I don't know. It just seems that ... I'm not sure ... I guess it's a double-ended sword. You could look at it as if people are in uniform they're going to be in that sort of set mode and they're going to do this better and they're going to be interested in learning, whereas people out of uniform might be a bit slacker and stuff. But I think they push it a bit far, like you get seen with your shirt out and it's an instant detention. Just stuff like that, I think is a bit over the top. (Jake)

There were some students however, who understood the value of uniform and how it set their school apart from many government schools and gave it the feel of an elite independent school. Nadine was student who placed a high premium on the appearance of students and what this could say about a school.

> We have a pretty strict uniform and they're pretty strict compared to other schools, and there's not many druggies compared to other schools. So you don't really see many people with slicked back blonde hair with black re-growth and eye make up everywhere. If you see someone like that you'd think 'Oooh what school do *they* go to?' (Nadine).

Discipline — The Dark Side of Schooling

For some students it was uniform that brought them face to face with the 'dark side' of the school. Within the context of the classroom, few teachers seemed to comment on a shirt not being tucked in; however, in the corridors students had to run the gauntlet of those members of staff who took most responsibility for discipline including year-level coordinators and Deputy Principals. Some of these members of staff loomed large in students' discussions and it was clear that several were very unpopular and considered to step beyond the bounds of what students felt was reasonable. When discussing these issues, students distinguished between the teachers and the administration. 'Administration' was a term used with reference to staff in the principal category, that is, the Principal and the two Deputy Principals, and sometimes students used this term in reference to the year-level coordinators. Miread, Daniel, Paul, and Stephen felt deeply about discipline and how it influenced the experience of school and, in particular, learning.

> **Daniel:** The principals, they run this school like clockwork.
>
> **Paul:** What does Mr Creasey [School Principal] do seriously?
>
> **Stephen:** I don't know, I don't see him do anything, he comes out of his office you know, every couple of days.
>
> **Miread:** Nah, Mr Smith [Deputy Principal] is very ...

Stephen: A bit of a Nazi ...

Miread: You can get abused, you can get called names, he'll grab you. He is just ... shocking.

Stephen: He's worse to the younger students.

Paul: As you get older, it gets better.

Miread: He takes it all out on them ... now that we're older, we just shrug it off ...

Miread: So, yeah.

Stephen: But the Year 7s and 8s get a lot of shit from him. He abuses them, and ...

Paul: He scares the crap out of them because they've never seen that sort of stuff.

Miread: Coming from primary school, where they're all nice ...

Stephen: Smith is horrible, he thinks it's just a student job thing, but it can really affect you emotionally some of the things he does. He'll tell you to do something, and two seconds later he'll yell at you to 'Come on, hurry up, hurry up.' But it's the way he yells.

Miread: See, he gets a lot of the bad jobs that the staff don't want to do, but he does it badly, like he treats everybody just below him. Even the staff ...

Stephen: He yells at the staff.

Miread: He degrades the younger teachers in front of us, he treats them like students — in front of us. And people sit there going 'Oh ... geez, feel sorry for them.'

GT: If you were Principal of the school what would you change?

Miread: I'd tell Smith where to go! I think I would just tell him that ... a lot. But I think he is one of the big problems with our school because his control is just, horrible. But apart from that, there isn't. Maybe just change the subjects a little bit to cater for others.

These students are concerned by what they see as 'horrible control' and the repercussions of this for younger students and younger staff. They describe a process that is degrading for junior staff, who are berated in front of students. Also with reference to younger students they are concerned because such students are identified as coming from schools where everyone is 'nice'. These students don't seem to challenge the need for discipline; they do, however, challenge the way in which this discipline is exercised by Mr Smith. This is also the case with Miread, who notes that his is a job that other staff do not want. Other students, however, mentioned Mr Smith with more sympathy. Ben and Aaron, who were completing Year 12 at the time of the interview, saw discipline in a different light.

GT: What do you think makes a school successful?

Ben: Probably it's dedicated faculty and probably Mr Smith. Like as much as people go on about him, I don't know, he's very — like sometimes dogmatic in his ways and stuff, but he knows what he — he gets there in the end. He kind of I suppose, keeps the school running smoothly and stuff. Mr Creasey is actually the Principal but he's kind of more quiet compared to Mr Smith.

Discipline for Learning

Students responded in a variety of ways to the type of authority represented by Mr Smith. However, there seemed to be a more uniform response to what made a good teacher good. For some, the issue was far from complicated. Nadine and Amy, for example, responded firmly in the following manner:

GT: What would you change if you were the Principal?

Nadine: I'd change all the teachers.

GT: What sort of teachers would you change?

Nadine: The ones that have no idea what's going on.

Amy: There are some teachers that can't control the class …

Nadine: A few teachers I can't stand.

GT: What is it about them?

Nadine: I have one teacher for two subjects, and she can't control the class and her marking is really inconsistent. Some of the accusations she makes against people. This guy was playing with his fly or something and she thought he was making sexual gestures.

Sebastian and Julian were interviewed after they had completed their Year 12 examinations. They reflected positively on their school.

Sebastian: We've had some absolutely great teachers and stuff, which has definitely made life a lot easier on us.

GT: What makes a teacher great?

Sebastian: I reckon someone you can relate to and someone who can kind of hold your attention, companionable, you know, someone who you are actually willing to associate with, so it kind of stops becoming a chore and kind of becomes interesting in itself, which is easier to do in a smaller class size I suppose. Like with literature this year, there's only about twenty-six/twenty-five people in the class and in our language class there's only about seven, so yes, we actually kind of got to get to know the other people in the class and the teachers. It's much better.

Julian: Otherwise the teachers we've had in the school, the good ones have been really good and the bad ones haven't been unbearable, so we've done pretty well as far as teachers go. The environment is good, the facilities are good too, no really horrible classrooms except in summer when some of the portables start to get a bit stuffy. They've put in air-conditioning now, in all portables, so it's good.

In a similar way, Ben and Aaron, who had also just completed their Year 12 examinations at the time of the interview, commented that teachers made a school successful.

Aaron: I think it's more the teachers that make it [school] successful you know. That's why you come here, because I mean if the teachers are good, then you get good results, get more students, and become successful.

Miread, Paul, Stephen, and Daniel were very open about their views of the teachers at the school. Whilst unhappy with the 'administration', they were generally happy with regard to the teachers. There were enough good teachers to compensate for those they regarded as 'dodgy'.

Miread: This school, a lot of the higher-up authorities like the Principal and everything like that, they ... I don't really like them. But when you go down to some of the younger teachers now — because we're getting in a lot of younger teachers — that's really good, because we can really relate to them and they treat us with a lot more respect than the others do. So it's good that they're getting younger teachers in ... which like ... I've noticed since Year 7 we had all ... people that shouldn't be doing their jobs, and now a lot of the teachers have improved, so that's good.

GT: It's improved because you've got new teachers rather than the teachers you have improving?

Miread: Yeah, yeah.

Stephen: Because that's what you need ...

Daniel: But also, as far as ... I can whinge about the admin till the cows come home, but the teaching staff themselves are very good as a rule.

Stephen: Most of them.

Daniel: You've always got ...

Paul: You've always got at least one ...

Stephen: If your teacher's dodgy, there's somebody else in the faculty that you can go to.

Miread: Yeah.

Stephen: Like if you've got a dodgy maths teacher this year.

Miread: Then you go to your last maths teacher.

Stephen: You've got other teachers in the area.

Daniel: And the teachers themselves, as a rule, are very good. They're always different — I'm not going to name names — but you know.

Paul: Of course, there's the horrid teachers ...

Daniel: There's some pretty dodgy teachers, but there's at least one or two that are really good in each faculty.

GT: And what is it about the administration?

Daniel: I would change the approach that a lot of the admin ... I s'pose takes. I know from personal experience, I work really well when I really like the teachers and respect them, and I work so I don't let them down rather than working because I have to. I know that I ... Ok, if I don't get on with the teacher it doesn't, I don't mesh with them, I'll still do it, but you don't have that same sort of flare and you don't really want to do well for that particular teacher. So I'd take a different sort of approach, rather than a 'If you do not do well at this, you'll spend the rest of your life in a gutter,' sort of approach, which is a very Leafy Suburbs College sort of sentence. And um ... and I would really take a more, a more easy-going approach. I realise that there are some sort of kids that need this one I s'pose, but I think that that is not going to change no matter what they do, whether it's an easy-going approach they're going to enjoy it more anyway. So I think that to do better I would change the approach towards the students and stuff.

Paul: The problem is the approach in Year 7 and 8 needs to be harder than the Years 10s 11s, etc. I think because this year we're realising that if we don't do well we're not going to be doing the jobs that we want to do, we're going to be doing some second-rate thing. But in Year 7 you're just like, 'Oh, don't give a shit, I've got like six years to learn. I can just stuff around for the next four years'.

Miread: I think Year 7, actually the whole course, should be a little bit more fun. Because in Year 7 and maybe Year 8 you are just stupid, you don't want to do work and the teachers treat you like dirt. And you know, Year 7's pretty, I mean it's a lead up to all the other years but it's not that crucial. And a lot of people don't enjoy it and because you're getting into the school and um ... yeah I reckon Year 7 especially should be more excursions, sort of things and stuff to get people into the work. Because I don't remember anything from Year 7 because it was just so boring. All I remember is terrorising teachers!

Daniel: And then you get to Year 10 and you're like, 'Oh I'm sorry I didn't mean that'.

Stephen: Oh yeah, they need to make the Year 7 course a bit harder so that we're prepared more for the Year 10 and 11. But they put a bit too much pressure on us. Like, right now, it's Year 10, we've got another two years to go for uni or TAFE [Technical and Further Education colleges] or whatever you're going to do and they're put so much pressure on you're thinking it is so crucial, that if you miss something or you don't do something you're just stuffed. And for teenagers especially between fourteen and seventeen it's a really hard time, and all that pressure can really get to you, and just make you freak out. I think they need to realise that.

Paul: They need to balance it more, I s'pose.

During this exchange, these students illustrate some of the tensions implicit in their expectation of the school. On the one hand, they are critical of the way junior students are treated and on the other hand, they consider how students, including themselves, can be 'stupid' at this stage of their lives. Miread comments that in her junior years she remembers 'terrorising teachers'. It remains unclear whether it is Miread or the teachers who are doing the terrorising. It is left to Daniel to clear up this ambiguity when he recognises the need to apologise to teachers for previous behaviour. Daniel also expresses the opinion that respect from teachers earns students' best efforts. He remains unconvinced that the Leafy Suburbs College approach works, even with students less motivated than himself and his friends.

Daniel: Well ... generally. I think streaming and people being where they want to be is really important because if you're not doing what you want to do, then it's not going to work, and that just links up to what I was saying before about teachers and working with teachers who you really want to work for and do what you want to do rather than what they make you do.

Stephen: But it's also um ... about the Principal thing ... Daniel saying when you have a teacher that you get on with and respect, you tend to do better because everything they tell you, you believe and you take in. Whereas over the last four years I've had so many dodgy teachers and um ... everything that they say you just sort of ignore or think you know, 'You're an idiot, you're talking crap.' Like I had a really shocking English teacher this year, and a bad French teacher and I've forgotten more things than I've learnt in the past three years.

GT: What makes a teacher bad?

Miread: Lack of respect.

Daniel: I don't think they appeal to you ... they rather say 'if you don't, you will fail and you will ...'

GT: So is that to do with their style?

Stephen: It's to do with the way they teach and their attitude.

Paul: There's also the, the problem with the teachers is that there's one of each type. There's the one like my English teacher, who had no control over the class and therefore we had no respect for her and we didn't want to do the work, and we'd be writing all this crap and you'd pull these amazing grades because you show a little bit of respect once in a while and you get it. But there's the other side of the scale, where there's the Mr. Geraldine, who's amazingly strict, he like hears the click of a pen and he just turns around and goes 'CHARLIE!'

GT: So is he a good teacher?

Paul: No, he's the other scale of bad.

Daniel: Some people say he's good.

Miread: See, I had him, he's bad because he's ... really quite excessive about it. It's almost amusing how ... we would sit there and do something and he'd just stare. But he got us such good marks, I mean some kids were nearly failing maths and they were getting B's and stuff.

Daniel: I remember him explaining table tennis to us once, like a military service. Like 'the ball must pass over THIS line at THIS particular point, if it DOESN'T make this particular POINT then ...' you know.

Miread: And you just think 'But I just want to play table tennis.'

Stephen: Well, um, I actually think of him as quite a bad teacher, I had him as a substitute once for maths and he is a maths teacher as well, and the way we work at this school, is, lots of people ... we help each other, and also ...

GT: You mean the students?

Paul: Yeah, the students.

Stephen: Yeah, part of school is not just the academic side, it's also the social. Forming relationships and friends and helping each other so that you're ready for the real world. And in his class, we were doing maths and previously they developed this theory of 'Three before me', but what it was was, try three things when you have a problem before asking the teacher. Mr Geraldine must have his philosophy of 'I teach you the work now you shut up and be quiet and do the work and we'll have a room full of silence throughout the class'.

Daniel: See, he'd be a brilliant one to learn ... See, when I have a problem I have to wait till the teacher gets all the way down the row.

Stephen: If you say one word, Mr Geraldine will crack the shits. If we have a problem in maths we discuss it with each other and he'd crack it, and because of this 'Three before me' thing we could talk back to him and say 'Hey we're doing this learning thing you suggested'. And he'd say 'Oh well, why don't you ask me?'. It's just crazy, his theory of silence just doesn't work. You need to discuss it.

Miread: Yeah.

Daniel:	Yeah, sometimes it'd work brilliantly one on one, but I don't think it's effective in a class room.
Stephen:	You need to talk with your peers and you need to work it out yourself.
Paul:	It also depends on what kind of class it is. If there is a maths and science class, then it's great to talk with one another because in the end you'll get the same answer anyway, and because you're talking with your peers you get it easier because they're explaining it to you. But in something like an English class or another class — where you can branch off on your own to create your own ideas and your own endings — talking in class kind of limits that a bit. So silence is more needed in the humanities subjects than in the mathematics ones.
Daniel:	Because really, you could talk the hind leg off a donkey in English.

There are a number of contradictions evident in this sequence, sometimes expressed by the same student. Daniel, for example, thinks a teacher who provides answers quickly is good; on the other hand, he sees the advantages in a system where students can talk and explore answers together. These are highly motivated students who were described as nerds. In this context, their insights are particularly interesting — what best facilitates learning varied, but respect seemed a critical aspect, both in terms of teachers respecting each other and the students and earning the respect of the students through their professionalism.

On Being a 'Good' School

The streets surrounding the sporting fields were gridlocked as what seemed like hundreds of cars stopped and opened their doors. Students converged from all directions and the sporting fields become instantaneously covered with colour. Each year the school athletics involved a particular theme as well as the house colours. This particular year students in togas decorated with green, red, blue, or yellow were in great number given the Olympic theme. Huddles of students gathered comparing outfits. It seemed a creative way of involving those with great as well as those with relatively limited athletic prowess.

The school's reputation was a recurring theme in conversations with parents, students, and teachers. This implied an assessment of the school relative to other schools. During discussions, most students compared Leafy Suburbs College to other government schools. A few students compared it to private schools. In itself, this seemed significant and indicated the possible context for school choice. Miread, Stephen, Daniel, and Paul consider Leafy Suburbs College relative to the government schools in the immediate vicinity. Miread has chosen to attend Alternative College the following year. This school has a reputation for a philosophy diametrically opposite to that of Leafy Suburbs College. No uniform, little discipline, a broader curriculum with an emphasis on what one teacher described as the 'arty-theatry-dramarey-creative stuff'. Many students who leave Leafy Suburbs College end up at Alternative College. Other schools are also mentioned including Suburbia College. In the past, some government schools were technical schools and initially, single-sex boys' schools. These schools catered to working-class boys who eventually went on to qualify in trades such as carpentry and plumbing. These existed in mainly working-class areas and relative to neighbourhood high schools, which were understood to cater for those who aspired to higher education or white-collar work, technical schools had a reputation for being tough. Such schools were phased out in the 1980s, but their reputation still lingers, as is evident in these students' comments.

GT: How do you think the school compares with others?

Stephen: I haven't been to other schools ... Some other schools just do shit-all and they have bad relationships with teachers and they don't learn anything and they get crap grades and they end up dropping out. So I think Leafy Suburbs College, along with its reputation, is quite good for achieving results. But like the others have said, if you're already achieving, you will continue to achieve, but if you are struggling, sometimes the teachers will tend to focus on you less if you need help. But overall, the school's quite good in comparison to other schools ... especially public schools considering we have limited funding. So yeah, we do quite well.

Miread: Um ... Ok. Well, I'll just give you an example. I went to ... I've been to a million Leafy Suburbs College Information] Nights and they sit there and say 'You will DO this and you will DO that' and 'You can do this for me' and it's all about what you can do for the school. I went to an Alternative College night, and they said 'How can we help you?' 'Why don't you come up to us and WE can help you to get good marks and we can help you to have fun and help you to be relaxed and if you have a problem come and see us, call me' and they're just relaxed. 'These are the subjects, we want to help you, we want to do this', and Leafy Suburbs is like 'You will do this for me'. And at Alternative I was confused! I thought, help me? You can do that? I haven't seen that for a while! And it's such a big difference, just the philosophy of the school. It's just so different. It's very ... I don't know, I totally suit Alternative a lot better because I don't like strong authority. And I think I can do things by myself and I like to work independently and I like to work with the teacher, I don't like to work under them. So I think Alternative will suit me better. So yeah, it's just the philosophy of the school, different schools have different philosophies. And like Suburbia — Suburbia is ... it's getting better, it used to be a lot worse than it is now ...

Stephen: It used to be a TECH school.

Miread: Yeah. So they're sort of trying to be like Leafy Suburbs, but I think they're sort of half way between Alternative and Leafy. Leafy and Alternative are like the two extremes and Suburbia's somewhere in the middle. But they don't really get the marks that Leafy does and they don't really have the freedom that Alternative does either. So a lot of people go in there and don't do as well. And that's like a lot of schools in the area.

Daniel: Leafy Suburbs College does work for me personally because you've got this fascist admin at the top who are pulling marks at us and then you've got these teachers who I really want to perform well for. And I think the teachers who appeal to you as friends, they really want to help you. And I do so well under them! So you've got them and the fascist administration, they're forcing the marks and they're [the teachers] making me want to work and it works really well. But if it's a good combination for me, but I know it doesn't work for everyone and I know schools like Alternative College are really brilliant. But then there's the Alternative Junior campus, and my mum's a teacher, and she used to teach at Alternative Junior and they gave her a nervous breakdown ... well, they didn't give her one but they almost did. She just refused to go back. She's now teaching at other schools, she's really nice and easy-going and the students took full advantage of that and just went raucous in the class room. And I don't think, I don't actually think the easy-going approach works on a junior level.

Miread: Oh yeah ... I agree with that.

Daniel: It's brilliant for senior, but not for junior.

Miread: See, my little sister goes to the Junior campus now because my parents thought that that school would be more suited to her and so they started her there instead of here. And she, it sounds like she's doing Ok. Like it's only year 7, you can't really tell, but I can see that the school is really different to our school and different to the senior campus. Because the kids take advantage of what they have and they just go crazy. It doesn't work when you're younger.

Paul: They don't have a work ethic. Leafy Suburbs creates one; between Year 7 and Year 10, it creates this whole 'You've got to do this', but once that's created, you can then go and leave to a place like Alternative and you've still got that ingrained thing that even though you don't have to do the work you're going to do it anyway, but not only do you want to but you've been taught for the last four years. It'd be nice to mix the both — the ingrained with the work ethic early on and then the senior ...

Daniel: The Leafy Suburbs junior method and the Alternative Senior method would be really good together. Because there's a point where you become ... well, I s'pose you grow up.

Miread: Yeah, mature enough to make your own decision.

These students recognise the benefits of a system they have criticised previously. Here, they contemplate why young students need to have a work ethic 'ingrained' into them. Such a work ethic is necessary in order to achieve academically in the senior year levels, and left to their own devices, young students 'just go crazy'. Daniel attests to the disadvantages of a system they describe as too lenient for junior students through his mother's teaching experience at Alternative. Miread uses the example of her younger sister to confirm Daniel's description of the school. Nonetheless, Miread is adamant about what makes this school superior to Leafy Suburbs College, why she has chosen to transfer to the school, and why it suits her better. She is a student who is independent, self-motivated, and who appreciates a student-centred approach. She describes her amazement at the shift in emphasis between Leafy Suburbs College and Alternative. Miread explains that at Alternative College teachers ask how they can help students achieve, while at Leafy Suburbs College, students are told what they need to do to fit in. The interviewees describe Leafy Suburbs College and Alternative College as extreme opposites and situate other schools, including Suburbia, between the two. Schools such as Suburbia do not achieve the noteworthy academic results for which Leafy Suburbs College is famous, nor do they offer the more relaxed atmosphere that makes Alternative College attractive. These students agree on a compromise. The ideal school combines the Leafy Suburbs College approach for junior students and the Alternative College approach for senior students. It is worth noting in this context that these students had not entered Year 11 at the time of the discussion. Students interviewed who had experienced Years 11 and 12 at Leafy Suburbs College commented on how teachers' attitudes toward them, including those of Mr Smith had altered as they entered the final years of their schooling. Perhaps Miread and her friends had yet to experience what made Leafy Suburbs College their ideal school.

Ben and Aaron had completed Year 11, and as discussed in Chapter 8, both students identified with the Jewish community. Ben's family had immigrated from South Africa. These boys reiterated that Leafy Suburbs College had a good reputation, but they tended to compare the school to private schools rather than neighbourhood government schools. Both boys had attended independent Jewish schools. Aaron had completed his primary schooling at one in Melbourne and chose to transfer to Leafy Suburbs College. Ben had attended such a school in Johannesburg.

GT: Oh, how do you think the school compares with others?

Ben: I think it's got a very good name. I'm not sure because I don't go to those schools, so I don't know what they're like, but yeah ... a lot of people try and queue up to get in here ... I've heard.

Aaron: I guess at the end of the day it's the results people get in Year 12 that gives schools their reputation. And I think, it's got a ... as I said before, the teachers, it's got a really diverse group of teachers which are always willing to put time in. And they've got really good facilities — the music's good, the sport's good, and you've got all the chess club and all that. But the music and sport, parents look for that kind of stuff if they're looking for a school for their kid.

Ben: I just wanted to say I think schools often gain a reputation quite easily. If you get a couple of incidents then you often ... the schools ... everyone boycotts it or something.

GT: This school is very popular, isn't it? Are your parents happy with you being here?

Ben: Yes, my parents are very happy.

Aaron: Yes, I know a few people who didn't get in and I thought, a lot of people showed up, my brother came here, so I just got in without much fuss, but I knew a few people that couldn't get in. The guy that went to Marysville Grammar, like he thought this school was much better than Marysville, so ...

Ben: I came from King David in South Africa, in Johannesburg, they've got a King David there and it's a big private school, like it's very big, it's probably even bigger than Leafy Suburbs, because it's got kind of a junior school onto it as well, so it's a very big school and when I came here I was originally going to go to Burstall Grammar ... But then also my parents had heard from people that this was one of the best public schools.

Ben and Aaron were well aware of the significance of school reputation. They described how a good reputation was hard won and easily lost.

Aaron: Because if you've got like a lot of fights and that you know, there's a couple, one that made the paper a few years ago about all these guys bashing up some girl or something down at the park from this school, but there's like, if there's too many of those articles you be a bit iffy about sending your kids here and it wouldn't make it a very successful school. Like Glenelg College [neighbourhood government school] already got a reputation for drugs and everything like that, so you know if you have a lot of fights and a lot of that sort of stuff, I reckon it would affect the school.

Ben: I just wanted to say I think schools often gain a reputation quite easily. If you get a couple of incidents then you often ... the schools ... everyone boycotts it or something.

GT: If you were the Principal what would you change?

Ben: Like what do you mean by change? In terms of school-wise or ...

GT: I mean about school, yes.

Aaron: As I'm not Principal ...

GT:	Maybe there's nothing to change.
Ben:	No, I've drawn a blank.

While some students were clear headed about the things they would change about their school, others were not. In the case of the latter, this may or may not reflect more contentment with the school.

Daniel:	The thing is, though, I think everybody should have access to all types of education. But I think the people that don't want to do that shouldn't have to be. Honestly, I think that this policy that everybody has to finish Year 12 thing ... well, yeah I see totally where they're coming from, it'd be a wonderful thing if everybody wanted to finish Year 12 and really wanted to be there, but I honestly think they should offer ... they should push apprenticeships and push things for the people that don't want to do academic stuff.

With this comment Daniel was able to summarise the debate that had been resurrected — the virtues of a common form of Year 12 certification. In 2002 the Victorian Government had introduced a new form of Year 12 assessment. The Victorian Certificate of Applied Learning (VCAL) would enable students to complete Year 12 without their curriculum being dominated by university gate-keeping functions. It is described (VCAA 2005) as 'hands-on learning' and recommended for students not intending to apply for a university place. Instead, it is a pathway from school toward work, an apprenticeship or further education at a Technical And Further Education (TAFE) college. Needless to say, Leafy Suburbs College had not introduced VCAL. In Daniel's mind, as with so many others, a university place is linked to the politics of performance, discipline instilled through seemingly irrelevant measures such as the wearing of ties and above all else, a like-mindedness premised on exclusion.

Chapter 12

Imagined Futures — Passion or Passionate Pragmatics?

> The act of imagination, as we have just seen, is a magical act. It is an incantation destined to make the object of one's thought, the thing one desires, appear in such a way that one can take possession of it. There is always, in that act, something of the imperious and the infantile, a refusal to take account of distance and difficulties.
>
> (Sartre 2004:125)

Perhaps becoming an adult requires that we let go of what Sartre identifies as the infantile and magical act of imagining you can achieve that which is distant. In the context of schooling, perhaps maturing is recognising that what you would like to become is too difficult. In the course of this study, I have been particularly interested to understand how students experience the school and how they see it facilitating the futures they imagine for themselves. This, in turn, brings into light the nature of the futures they imagine. Leafy Suburbs College is a school that promises success, defined as good academic results, in turn situated in relation to university entry. In this context, students are given permission to imagine futures linked to prestigious careers. However, for some, such careers stand in contrast to what they are really passionate about. Jake, the charismatic piano player, was illustrative of this. He was a stand-out musician who also identified sport as central to his identity. He described how many people assumed that being 'sporty' and being a 'muso' were incompatible. For his final years of schooling, he had combined Physical Education, Biology, Music, and Mathematics. He contrasted his subject choices to those of 'nerds' who he described as doing 'more sciency' subjects including Chemistry and Physics. He also contrasted his choices with those of other 'musos' who included 'arty' subjects like Visual Communication and Design and Studio Arts in their curriculum.

How did Jake imagine his future? He was interviewed near the end of Year 11 when he was contemplating the last year of his schooling and where this would eventually lead him. He stated that after Year 12 he was considering two options: going to university to undertake study in an alternative health area (massage and acupuncture) or working in a trade such as carpentry. The divergent nature of these alternatives surprised me, but Jake was straightforward in his explanation. Alternative medicine flowed naturally from his interest in sport and therefore the body. This was why he was undertaking related subjects such as biology and physical education. He stated, 'I think people these days are sort of looking for alternative things rather than going to doctors and getting pills'. A trade would give him the opportunity to work outdoors, which he felt he would enjoy. However, he commented that he 'could get bored with doing a trade. I s'pose because you'd be doing the same thing over and over'. The alternative health industry provided the opportunity for what he termed 'constant learning'. He totally dismissed music as a career option.

> Yeah, I love it [music], but I'm not going to do it because ... I'm still going to play gigs for sure and still practice ... but it's not the right sort of ... if I had my own way I'd do music, but to do the things I love doing like surfing and windsurfing and water-skiing and skiing down slopes and stuff, I need that sort of money, and ... music doesn't really cut it ... but I'm still going to play gigs and stuff for sure, music's one of the biggest parts of my life definitely. (Jake)

Jake imagined his future through three interrelated priorities — his love of music, his career preference, and the need for the type of financial security that would support expensive recreational activities. In his balancing of priorities he was clear that music would not provide him with the necessary financial security. He was also clear that financial security was something he would not forgo. In so doing, Jake arguably suspended his primary identification, that of 'muso'. While he 'loves' music and will always 'practice' and 'play gigs', music is not part of his imagined professional future. In some ways this exemplifies sophisticated identity work, the balancing of a range of competing priorities and an adept shape-shifting capacity. He is comfortable with being both 'muso' and 'sporty' even if these choices appear counterintuitive. He is comfortable with being either a carpenter or someone who works in the alternative health industry, again alternatives that seem to grow out of disparate interests.

So while Jake's primary and most public identification at school was being a 'muso' and this coincided with his passion, his imagined future related to very different fields of endeavour. In the future, Jake imagined his 'muso' identity would be relegated to his private sphere. The division Jake makes here between passion and pragmatics was reiterated by other students and needs to be considered in relation to schooling more generally. Are we teaching passionate pragmatics rather than a pragmatics of passion?

Fiddling with Success

Sebastian and Julian were also identified as 'musos'. Their style was in keeping with what they described as 'bohemian' and in contrast to Jake it was difficult to imagine them surfing or skiing. Instead, they spent time in cafés exchanging opinions about music and politics. They were philosophical and analytical in their approach. The set of opinions they expressed about the virtues of school uniform and the necessity for structure and discipline as a means whereby students achieved good academic results did not appear compatible with their dress and hairstyles, which projected countercultural traits. They had applied to do postschool courses in graphics and multimedia design. Sebastian explained:

> I really enjoy the Art kind of stuff. I like just being able to fiddle. I like the whole tactile side of just being able to draw and fiddle around and stuff. (Sebastian)

This choice fitted in with what Jake had described as the 'arty' subjects 'musos' liked. Yet in their last year of schooling, Julian and Sebastian had taken music subjects, double mathematics, and a Language Other Than English. Like Jake, they had studied music at school, but were not intending to continue studying in this area, despite the central place music occupied in their self-identification.

GT: But you're both into music?

Sebastian: Yes.

GT: But that's not something you're taking further?

Sebastian: No, because we've heard all these horror stories about how hard a muso's life is, although if we do get into a course this year, we're going to defer for a year and then see, have a crack at making it in the music industry and you know …

Julian: Yes, or not so much, we're just going to try and get some stuff recorded and fiddle around and see what happens, see if it works, and if it works maybe keep going with it on the side because I mean whatever happens with it, we're definitely still going to be doing music as a hobby or whatever just because we enjoy it so much and you know we've got each other. We can kind of jam with each other and all of that.

Sebastian: Yes, that's really good.

Julian: Well, it's hard to make enough money, get enough solid employment solely as a muso to kind of subsist within ...

Sebastian: There's no constant employment, there's no constant money source. You've got to ...

Julian: Unless you get a residency or something which is like a stable gig every month or so and you get really lucky and get famous and discovered and then supposedly the money just rolls in, but either way, it's supposedly a very stressful lifestyle, constant demands.

Sebastian: Yes, deadlines is also something we're not good at and stress and all that so ...

Julian: Musos are not all that great at meeting deadlines or being organised.

GT: But how will you do graphics? How do you make your money in the real world?

Sebastian: I'm thinking of a couple of friends of ours, a guy in Year 12 this year has started up his own design thing over the Internet and he's done a couple of — he's worked for his mates and for a couple of people he's met on the Internet and he's looking at getting us and a couple of other people from the Year-level in, and starting up a proper graphics company. He's already made a bit of money just by himself. He's made a couple of thousand dollars just through kind of messing around.

Julian: It's a good industry, but it's very, very competitive. A lot out there, a large talent base and all the training and stuff that you get these days just means that there's even more competition, so it's demanding, but it's probably worth it. If that fails, we'll probably try and work our way into a graphics company. As a long-term goal, I'm trying to get into animation.

These boys are pessimistic about the possibility of sustaining themselves through music — they have heard the 'horror' stories. This is despite the fact that between them, they play seven instruments and their music teacher described how their ensemble achieved the top exam results for the state. Like Jake, they describe how music will remain both central and peripheral in their imagined futures.

Julian and Sebastian are concerned to minimise stress in their lives and during our discussion described how graphics, whilst demanding and competitive, was 'worth it'. This was a calculated estimation that situated music by comparison, as not 'worth it'. This theme related to worthwhile stress was strong in their responses to a number of issues. The strict uniform code and discipline at the school was worth the likelihood of good academic results. In this context, they contrasted Leafy Suburbs College to the neighbourhood school with no uniform requirements, liberal discipline policies, and lower academic results. The amount of schoolwork they did allowed them to achieve A grades however, working toward A+ grades was not worth the stress. In terms of their own ambitions, they wanted work that would afford them a lifestyle they enjoyed. Like Jake, they wanted the opportunity to do things that were meaningful to them, rather than find meaning in what they were expected to do.

GT:	And what's your idea of success in your own life?
Sebastian:	Whatever it is I have to be enjoying it. That's about it to be able to get the enjoyment I want out of it and still survive.
Julian:	Yes, I think to be able to — yes, relax and not have to stress too much. You know find some sort of job or occupation even if it was you know waiting tables or something, where I could exist comfortably without having to kind of panic and stress, so I can have time to stuff …
Sebastian:	To be able to live within your means.
GT:	And stuff that you need?
Sebastian:	Oh, music, friends, you know, drawing, whatever.
Julian:	Yeah, those are the types of things we find enjoyable, our various hobbies and things.
GT:	And do you reckon if you didn't have those other interests, general rather than rhetorical question — do you think that's what makes you happy with that definition of a successful life.
Sebastian:	I think so because if I didn't have them, I would probably define success as something completely different and if I didn't have that sort of release, then it would probably be something unattainable.
Julian:	Yeah, and even that sort of mind-set, you know to be able to enjoy like small things. Just to be able to kind of realise yeah, I have to go to school, I have to you know do whatever but I can still kind of enjoy myself, have a cup of coffee, you know talk to friends without kind of being too far one way or the other.
Sebastian:	Yeah, if you don't have that — if you are too far academic, well there's not all that much to sustain you, so I think that overwork is not healthy at all you know, so if you don't have any release then something is not right, you've got to have some sort of balance there. If you just keep working for work's sake, then eventually you're going to self-destruct because eventually you're going to either run out of work or be unable to work.
Julian:	And either way you're not happy.
Sebastian:	Something is going to collapse, so if success is work then I want no part of it.
GT:	But you're obviously keen on working, you're mainly saying that.

> **Sebastian:** We're willing to work because you know it's the only way we can kind of maintain the lifestyle which we want to enjoy. Frustratingly enough, you do need money, to be able to you know go out and meet friends and all that.
>
> **Julian:** You do need to work to get money, so we are willing to do what we have to do to sustain ourselves. Sometimes reluctantly.

Sebastian and Julian do not see themselves as conforming. Instead, they have a view of success that is tied to a balance between work and lifestyle. Nonetheless, their reluctance to be driven still yields them A grades. Their artwork and their musicianship (and their responses to my questions) illustrate that they are deeply thoughtful and exceptionally talented students. Teachers view them in this light and other students are in awe of them. By their own admission, arrogance is something they need to keep in check. Perhaps the ease with which they are able to achieve A grades provides them with an opportunity to create the balance they hold so dear. Other students need to work harder for as much or even less.

Focused on Being Middling

Aaron and Ben were also described as 'musos'. Like Jake, these students were interviewed as they neared the end of Year 11. They were talented musicians and Ben, in particular, was identified within the school in relation to his saxophone-playing persona. However, neither Aaron nor Ben stuck in the public imagination in the same way as Sebastian, Julian, or Jake. By their own description, they were in the 'middle group' — between the popular kids and the nerds. Aaron aspired to enter engineering and accordingly had chosen the science stream. Ben wished to study law and had chosen to do English Literature, Music Methods, and Chemistry. These students had strong ties with the Jewish community and constructed themselves as fitting into a range of groups and activities without being extreme about any of them. Their involvement with the Jewish community, as with their music, sport, and socialising generally, was sensible rather than extreme.

> **GT:** Why law?
>
> **Ben:** I don't know. I've been interested in it like since I was like seven years old and I don't know, I've just always had an interest in it, interest in the law and anything like that.
>
> **Aaron:** I'll probably do some sort of engineering perhaps. Yes, I don't know — I enjoy electronics stuff, and also because I also like a lot of music and stuff, so maybe even perhaps if it's like stage engineering or something for productions or something. I'm not 100% sure.
>
> **Ben:** Well, I think if you want to get the most out of school, you can't just be a complete study freak all the time. You have to have a bit of a social life and

	obviously school is like — one of the main aspects of it is I suppose to make new friends and stuff — I mean when you're going to school.
Aaron:	Yeah, you have to work hard, but yeah, you also have to go out sometimes. My brother said he didn't go out at all during his VCE year and he said it was the worst mistake he's ever made. He said, you know, it got really monotonous and you really, like if you've got somewhere to be, then you look forward to studying because you know at the end of it you know you're going out and stuff, so you've got to still work out as well.
GT:	Did he do well?
Aaron:	Yes, he did pretty well. He mucked up his English exam, which he didn't do too well, but apart from that yes, and he still got a pretty high ENTER score, so he didn't do too bad, but he said he could have done much better if he went out a bit. He just stayed home the whole time.
Ben:	I suppose probably students with a goal, if you know what you want to do or if you've got something that you want to achieve, I suppose you can work towards it and stuff because otherwise you just I suppose — like you don't have much, not much incentive to do any work and stuff. Got bored.

There was no self-doubt in the voices of Ben or Aaron, nor was there the self-invention that characterised Sebastian and Julian. They shared the same matter-of-fact approach to life that Jake had, but in seemingly more conventional ways. Their high aspirations fitted in with family expectations. Aaron's family had recently immigrated from South Africa and Leafy Suburbs College was recommended by Australian contacts prior to arrival. Aaron commented;

> ... my parents had heard from people that this was one of the best public schools, and also because we found a place in the area, a house in the area, so it would be easier probably to come here and so yes, that's why I came here. (Aaron)

It seems that for Aaron and Ben, school was about facilitating imagined futures in straightforward ways. It was almost like a contract — do the right thing and the right thing would happen in return.

Coincidentally, I bumped into Ben at a local shopping centre after he had received his Year 12 results. His score was good enough to enter Law but at a less prestigious university than the one he wanted to attend. He was debating whether or not to accept this place or enter Arts at the more prestigious university and seek a transfer to Law at a later stage. He chose the bird in the hand.

Marrying Millionaires and Buying Lottery Tickets

Anna, Sophia, and Lucy wanted to finish school, but did not aspire to enter university. The subjects they had selected reflected ambitions more modest than those of other interviewees. As discussed in Chapter 7, these girls seemed to me the least engaged with school, both in terms of academic work and extracurricular activities. They were identified as 'wogs' by the students who suggested I interview them, but did not refer to themselves in this way. They were difficult to interview. They were polite and attentive, but nonetheless, very circumspect about their lives, experiences, and feelings. This was Lucy's last day at the school. She aspired to hospitality and as a consequence was leaving Leafy Suburbs College to attend Alternative College the following year. Alternative College offered a range of vocationally orientated subjects specific to her area of interest.

GT: What do you see yourselves doing?

Sophia: Interior design or visual merchandiser …

GT: What's a visual merchandiser? I've never heard of that!

Sophia: Um … like setting up shop fronts and stuff, setting up shops.

GT: And you've made your mind up?

Sophia: Yeah.

GT: What do you need for that?

Sophia: English, Graphics, Studio Arts is an option and nothing else really … a bit of maths and that's about it.

GT: And hospitality? What does that involve?

Lucy: A lot of different things. It's everything to do with people and tourism; you can do things like that. And, cooking and working in restaurants and being a hotel manager just, working in those areas.

GT: And you're looking forward to that?

Lucy: Yeah.

GT: What made you choose that?

Lucy: I don't know because I'm always changing my mind about what I wanted to do, and one day I decided to do that, and it's stuck. I'm a bit excited but I don't know totally …

GT: And what about you Sophia? Why did you choose?

Sophia: I don't know, I like setting up things and colours and stuff.

GT: Oh good …

Anna: I'm still undecided, I don't exactly know what it is exactly that I want to do once I leave. Maybe something to do with tourism or business, I really don't know, it depends how I go, I guess.

GT: And you all see yourselves finishing school?

Anna:	Yeah,
Sophia:	Yeah.
GT:	Looking forward to the next two years?
Anna:	No! It's going to be hard, too much work.
Sophia:	Stressful.
GT:	Stressful? So you're going into Year 11 next year and you're all scared. Is everyone like that do you think?
Anna:	Some people have done Year 11 subjects this year, so they know … they've got a slight idea, and it's like they've already done their Year 11 subject. It's just scary — VCE.
Sophia:	I think it depends on how you go in Year 10, more than other year levels, like if you're going well or if you're failing. It just depends on that …

By their own description, Sophia and Anna were not looking forward to Year 11, which they anticipated being 'stressful'. For them, VCE was 'scary'. According to them, this was in part due to the fact that unlike many of their peers who were already doing accelerated programs, they were unaware of what was involved.

All three girls wanted to get married and have children in the future. Anna explained that currently, 'It's more about boyfriends and what I'm wearing on the weekend and stuff' that preoccupied her. I asked what they saw themselves doing in ten years' time, when they would be twenty-five years of age.

Lucy:	Wouldn't have a clue.
	Hopefully have a job, a partner, friends, wealthy, living by myself with my friends … in Toorak [an extremely wealthy Melbourne suburb]! (laughs). Nah, I don't know!
GT:	Is that what you'd like to be doing?
Anna:	I want to be rich!
GT:	So how do you think you'll get rich?
Anna:	Um … marry a millionaire! (laughs) That's my plan … when I'm old enough to marry.
GT:	What about you two? What do you reckon you'll be doing in ten year's time?
Sophia:	Travelling, hopefully wealthy as well.
GT:	You want to be wealthy too; how are you going to get wealthy? There are not that many millionaires around!
Anna:	We'll find two!

While it would be easy to consider these girls as simply preening and pining for the wealthy husbands manufactured through soap operas, this view of them is worthy of reconsideration. Anna was the only student interviewed who was involved intensively in part-time work on the weekends. She lived with her mother who was a sole parent. Sophia's family were hard-working immigrants. Her apprehension regarding scholastic success may have been tied up with wishing to live up to her parents' expectations. Lucy said least during the interview. She was leaving Leafy Suburbs College to begin at her third secondary school in as many years. These factors brought to my mind a range of scenarios less comfortable than those I imagined for other interviewees. Perhaps knowing that there is less likelihood of easy success makes you wish for the less probable — a bit like investing hope in a lottery ticket.

Imagined Futures

I have been particularly interested in understanding how students experience the school and how they see it facilitating the futures they imagine for themselves. This, in turn, brings into light the nature of the futures they imagine. During my discussions with Miread, Stephen, Daniel, and Paul, such issues were at the forefront of these students' minds, given the counselling process being undertaken toward their final subject selection at the time of the interview. This was a critical step in negotiating the best results for the students (and the school). And as indicated by some of their comments, this brought into stark relief the tension between different understandings of the worth and purpose of education. Each of these students was sceptical about aspects of the school culture, yet each had negotiated a different way of facilitating their imagined futures in relation to this culture.

Miread offered the most extreme position by choosing to leave the school at the end of the year. During the interview, Miread described how she aspired to do something she considered socially worthwhile. She identified teaching because social work was 'too depressing'. Miread explained that for her the nature of the work, rather than the remuneration, was most significant. Miread believed that Leafy Suburbs College would provide her with a better chance of attaining a high score. Yet she described how she was willing to risk leaving the school. Her risk-management strategy was linked to the estimation of her worth as an independent learner and the importance she attached to studying the subjects of most interest to her. Miread also described the way her brother who was identified as a 'jock', had been treated by the school. Being an A+ student who was asked to stay, meant that Miread had the power to choose, unlike her brother. Her decision to leave, albeit risky, seemed laced with retribution against the school, as well as loyalty to the students, like her brother, who in her terms didn't fit the system and got 'shuffled out'.

Stephen had a very different response to the school to that expressed by Miread. Having entered the school through the accelerated learning program, he was obliged to enrol in specific subjects. With only one subject choice available to him, he elected a Language Other Than English which he thought would give him some further options but also facilitate a high end of school score. Stephen saw himself entering, either medicine or engineering, university courses commensurate with the score he imagined he would achieve. This was almost a fait accompli — something that had its own momentum that would sweep him along. Like his participation in the accelerated program, it was a matter of entering into the most difficult thing possible rather than doing something you were passionate about.

Paul was a very keen musician and although he was interested in the same subjects as Miread, stated he would not forgo the school music program in order to do his preferred subjects at another school. A straight humanities student, he aspired to do a double degree in law and music. This was his way of reconciling his love of music and his belief that this would not lead to a comfortable lifestyle in the future.

Daniel, like Miread, aspired to do something he considered socially worthwhile.

> I don't want to do something that I'm only doing because it gives me a paycheck, I want to do something — I would actually rather be poor and doing what I want than have lots of money and doing what I don't like. And ... I kind of want to be remembered! (Daniel).

He saw himself studying for many years to come, perhaps history at a postgraduate level. He aspired to humanitarian, diplomatic, or political work. He mentioned the United Nations, humanitarian aid programs, or becoming a politician specifically. Like Paul and Miread, he wanted to do some subjects that were not available at the school. Unlike Miread, he chose to stay at the school and compromised his subject choices instead.

Students negotiate and compromise between the cultures they bring with them to school, those available to them, and those to which they aspire. Life is about deciding between available options and school is an important part of learning this. Miread, for example, decided to leave the school. She was far from romantic about what was at stake. As a former 'blonde' girl, she was deeply aware of the stigma and limitations associated with this label. Her refusal to stay was coloured by her brother's experience and her deep sense that the school did not value all students equally. This had been a lesson in life. She had a sense that doing it her way was going to be tough. Paul was far more strategic. Despite being a 'muso', he was not part of the 'popular' group and had already decided that his love of music would not translate into the lifestyle offered through a law degree.

His compromise was to do both and to name music as the hobby and law as the career. A law/music double degree reflected his vacillation between the 'musos' and 'nerds'. Stephen decided that he would tackle the most prestigious option available to him. While slipping between the 'Asian' and 'nerd' subcultures, he was also marginal to these. In part this was due to his participation in the school theatre program, but more significant was his decision to come out as gay. This gave him kudos amongst some students, but also defined him as Other. More to the point, his sexuality also had a price. During the interview, he spent much time describing what he considered to be overtly homophobic bullying he had experienced from a member of staff and some of the 'jocks'. He also described the complex set of relations that surrounded the support he could seek and receive from a gay teacher on staff. Arguably, Stephen was the most vulnerable of these four students and as such may have already understood the imperative to succeed in mainstream terms as a form of limited protection. Daniel was in a space between 'nerd' and 'popular kid'. A good-looking and articulate student with highly developed social skills, he combined his studies with a social life that was not the usual parties that the 'popular' kids attended. Subsequent to the interview, Daniel excelled in Year 11, spent two months in Europe on an exchange program and was being considered for the School Captaincy as he entered his final year of school. He was debating whether or not to accept this position given the connotations of co-option with which it was associated in his mind. Yet it was clearly tempting and possibly illustrative of his ambition 'to be remembered'.

Each of these students was clear about their futures and the central role of education within these. They were all clear that Leafy Suburbs College would assist them to achieve entry to university. However, they were all sceptical about aspects of the school culture. Because of this scepticism, these students were left with the task of mediating a sense of self that reconciled their imagined futures with their understandings of a school culture that for them symbolised an unjust system. This mediation of identity drew on their experiences of student school subcultures in various ways.

Jake was interviewed as he approached his final year of schooling. He went on to complete Year 12 and achieved results that were not high enough for him to enter the university course of his choice (sport and outdoor recreation). He did receive a place in a university course, which he had not initially chosen. He deferred for six months to work as a landscape gardener in a family business. He began his course and left after two months to return to work. After a year working, he applied to join a university conservatorium on the basis of audition and was waiting on the results of his audition. Perhaps, weighing up passion and pragmatics appropriately relies on life, not school experience.

Chapter 13

Identity as Academic Liability

The Victorian students who gain places at the two most elite universities, disproportionately come from elite independent and Catholic schools. Their attendance at such schools is readily linked to their parents' high socioeconomic status (Teese and Polesel 2003; Birrell et al. 2002; Edwards, Birrell, and Smith 2005). Leafy Suburbs College has a school population that is less straightforward. Many of its students do not share the backgrounds of their peers attending elite nongovernment schools. Many were born overseas. Many are the children of the so-called second generation those born in Australia to post–World War II immigrants. These are students who cannot communicate with their grandparents because they no longer share a common language. Many come from single-parent households. A significant number qualify for government maintenance allowances. Some of these students were described by teachers interviewed as 'Aussie battlers', those who do not share the middle-class ethos that dominates the school. Yet the majority of the students who attend Leafy Suburbs College complete Year 12 and gain a university place, including at the two most elite Victorian universities. Leafy Suburbs College was chosen for this study because of the diversity within the student population and the fact that this complicated the somewhat straightforward link between good VCE results and elite private schools. The intention has been to explore what happens at a government school with a diverse student population, where students access what is not automatically assumed as theirs. Rather than consider this issue in the context of debates about effective schooling or effective teaching, the aim has been to explore how students from various backgrounds experience the every day of their schooling. Most consideration has been given to how students reconcile who they are and who they want to become by mediating the dominant culture of the school and the various student subcultures. The argument has been made (Ball et al. 2002) that for students for whom university education is not a pre-given, such as those from ethnic minorities or the working-class, choice is risky because it is tied up with becoming something unfamiliar. As such, choice is multilayered and pragmatic, but also imbued with the nonrational and the cultural. In this sense, this study has been an exploration of students' identity choices as these relate to their imagined futures and the processes of identification that occur within a school that has been shaped as successful by market processes.

Students and staff involved in the study identified student subgroups that existed within the school. In turn, each of these was linked to academic success. The 'nerds' were most notably associated with academic success, particularly in 'sciencey' subjects. 'Jocks' or sporty kids were associated with athleticism and placed at the other end of the academic spectrum. In the case of the 'musos', they were primarily considered in relation to their musical aptitude; however, this could coincide with academic prowess or not. Most commonly, the referent for these labels was masculine behaviour. 'The wogs' were students who had an association with migration, most commonly from Europe. Their dress was modelled on that of 'gangster rappers' and they adopted particular mannerisms, accents, and language codes. They were ostracised, tough, and not commonly associated with strong academic achievement. Girls were described as 'female versions' of wog boys. In the case of some subcultures, however, the girls complimented rather than imitated the boys. In the case of the 'blonde' girls, they were more likely to look on while 'their boys', the jocks, played sport, than participate themselves. Yet they were formidable because of their capacity to intimidate other students through their association with this group of boys. In the case of 'nerds', girls and boys behaved in similar ways, but along parallel and nonintersecting pathways. This was also the case with the students others referred to as 'the Asians', and 'the Russians', groups whose membership overlapped significantly with the high academic achievers. While many girls were involved in the school music program, few were lauded as bone fide 'musos' in the same way as the charismatic boys who played lead saxophone, trumpet, piano, and drums. For these boys, theirs was an induction into a well-established culture performed, practised, privileged at the school, as in society more generally.

These were the prominent subcultures described by interviewees. Of the subcultures named, some remain 'unvoiced' in this text. The students who were relatively newly arrived immigrants — the so-called 'Asians' and 'Russians' — did not actively participate in this study. Similarly, the 'wog' boys and students who identified as Goths or punks were not interviewed. Instead, such groups were talked about by others and observed. The perspectives represented here are determined by my construction of those individuals who allowed me into their lives. Nonetheless, there is a sense of some of the issues at play in a school like Leafy Suburbs College at a broader level. Additionally, there is a sense of how a school such as this, an elite public school, plays at being a counterpublic in the way described by Weis and Fine (2001). Is it possible for a school, which is privileged relative to other public schools, to be constructed as having radical potential, particularly when its pedagogies of performance and politics of enrolment are arguably nontransformative and undemocratic? I wish to argue, somewhat counterintuitively, that this is the case. In Victoria, few government schools succeed in disrupting the seemingly natural conduit between elite independent and Catholic schools and elite universities. A school like Leafy Suburbs College has to do more with less in order to get its students over the line and by doing this, complicate the mix of students who enter elite universities. There are limited resources and therefore limited options. Leafy Suburbs College has decided to present as an academic school and in order to do so successfully, has to offer a limited range of subjects. These need to be taught in a way that caters for those students who are most likely to achieve. As one of the students interviewed commented, the school helps those students who need help the least and tends to offer less help to the others.

I have argued that its status as a 'pretend private' school makes Leafy Suburbs College an 'in-between' place — one shaped by both privilege and burden. Once enrolled, students have a better chance of making it to university; however, this involves hard work and the type of compromise that allows them to somehow merge with the persona of the 'good student', which is at such a high premium at the school. This type of 'good student' is produced through a range of exclusionary practices and harsh disciplinary measures. Nonetheless, I would like to argue that students, to varying degrees, allow themselves to be captured as 'good students'. In this way, they are complicit rather than acted upon, and the intention has been to consider some students in detail in order to provide insights into this process. This is an exploration of the compromises made and not made along the way to becoming a 'good student' and the motivations behind such compromises.

Students interviewed seemed to have little personal investment in the subcultures they named. Identities belonged to others and not to them. Identifying what it meant to be a 'nerd' or 'muso' was relevant to the extent that students defined the associated stereotype and then described how they did not fit the stereotype. Jake was not the stereotypical 'muso' because he played sport. Yet equally, he was not the stereotypical 'jock' because he played music. Nicole performed the 'blonde' girl, yet on closer examination she had chosen an academically rigorous curriculum, did little socialising outside of school, and maintained her subgroup standing through relentless intrigue at the school cafeteria. Ben and Aaron revelled in being 'middling'. They were 'muso', 'nerd', 'sporty', 'social', and 'Jewish', all in moderation. This was another way of staying between the range of subgroups that existed within the school rather than existing within any one of them. The so-called 'wog' girls made little mention of this group. Instead, they confirmed their disengagement with a school culture that seemed to wash over them failing to include them in any significant way. In the case of Dimitri, the school confirmed his belonging by attempting to exclude him. Miread, on the other hand, wanted to leave despite being asked to stay — an act of defiance, a statement that she was not what the school wanted her to be. Paul, Daniel, and Stephen qualified themselves as nerds — they excelled academically but retained an edge. Paul was committed to music yet wanted to do law. Daniel was debating whether to take on the School Captaincy. He was contemplating whether or not he could remain critical of a school culture he thought was domineering if he accepted a leadership position. He wondered whether leadership would make him complicit or give him an opportunity to instigate change. Perhaps more so than Daniel, with his overt interest in politics, Stephen understood power. As a gay student who had experienced bullying, lack of protection from mainstream structures, and limited support from gay teachers, he had decided to look after himself by becoming the best he could be within traditional frames of reference. Sebastian and Julian provided the most dramatic insights into a form of identity as denial. They were the consummate shapeshifters. Their identity relied on not having one — instead they 'synthesised self' — moved between categories, mutated through pastiche, playful irony, and illusion. Above all else, they wished to remain relaxed. They had understood the benefits of gaining B+'s and A's without stress, relative to gaining A+s with stress. The former allowed them to move between 'nerd', 'muso', and 'punk' and to confirm an identity that relied on avoiding being named as something.

These students provided clear insights into their school and the ambivalent place it occupied as a 'pretend private' school. They enjoyed what made it better than other government schools in their eyes, and simultaneously adopted the mantle of underdogs relative to students who attended elite nongovernment schools. They took pride in being able to compete favourably with significantly less. Yet these students were well aware of the cost of this success. There were strong statements from many students, including those most successful, describing what they thought was wrong with their school. However, few students chose to leave the school of their own volition. Then again, choice is not equally available or benign in its consequences. Miread had chosen to leave Leafy Suburbs College against the counsel of her teachers, but as an A+ student who resiled from the prevailing school culture, she felt that she could succeed at Alternative College because she was an independent learner. Dimitri, on the other hand, had chosen to stay at the school despite feeling that staff were attempting to push him out. He was disengaged and academically unsuccessful. Yet Dimitri was ambitious and had a sense that he could achieve. His act of staying was as much an act of resistance as Miread's choice to leave.

Just as the students were aware of the costs of being at a 'pretend private' school, so too did parents. For those interviewed, it was a matter of getting their children into the best school available to them. Given the common assumption that excellence is linked to price, these parents felt that Leafy Suburbs College was as good as they would get for the money invested. Many had worked hard to gain their children a place, either through astute property buying, investment in tuition, or sheer persistence. Informal discussion with parents illustrated an assumption that things would be more straightforward if they could afford to pay the fees demanded by elite private schools. In this way, despite the privilege of enrolment, Leafy Suburbs College was the fall-back position — the school you enrolled your child in when you couldn't afford your school of choice.

The same feeling was not in evidence amongst the staff. The staff interviewed voiced a deep commitment to public education. It was evident working at the school that teachers were dedicated to the school and the students. The Principal was proud that the school had achieved a ranking for staff satisfaction on a recent survey, which was one of the highest for the state. Clearly, teachers were happy to be at Leafy Suburbs College and why not? Many had their own children at the school and compared to other government schools, it was better resourced, and considered to have fewer 'problem' students. While some teachers voiced their concerns about the politics of enrolment and harsh discipline that excluded some groups of students, they were nonetheless aware of how such policies made teaching easier and more satisfying. As one interviewee commented:

> If I had to struggle with classroom management, potential violence out in the corridor or in the yard, or bickering and squabbling like I'm aware that's happened in other schools, for example, when they've had to meld or something like that — if I had to teach in an environment like that, I wouldn't bother.

For another teacher, it was a case of 'classing up' by being at Leafy Suburbs College.

> I feel a bit alienated from these people sometimes. Sometimes I think the kids here are a bit precious, and I'll have to say to them well, the world is not always like that and you're

not always given these things. You don't always have two parents and you know all this sort of stuff, so often I'll give them a bit of a reality check. Because I shifted from lower working-class to middle-class over the last thirty years, I'm sort of living in the middle-class now, the way I'm living now is sort of middle-class and I'm teaching at that level — I'd have to go backwards, and that would be interesting I think, I would have no worries about living and working in working-class suburbs.

The imposing brick fence opens onto large and well-cared-for school gardens and playing fields. The lights shine through the fancy cut glass of the large windows that frame the dining hall where the boarders sit for their evening meal. The courtyard circles a water feature where students from a number of schools congregate. Most clusters of students surround a teacher with clipboard in hand. The students, all wearing school uniform, are engrossed in last-minute preparations for the night's round of debates. Leafy Suburbs College is the only nonselective government school competing in this region of the state debating competition. Like the school, we are visiting for tonight's round of debating; most of the others are prestigious ones with some of the best VCE results for the state. Elite Catholic and independent schools, including some Jewish schools, are amongst those represented. There is a mixture of single-sex boys' and girls' schools and coeducational schools. Each school is familiar to those in attendance through uniforms with their distinctive colours and crests. There are some parents in attendance along with the volunteer adjudicators for the night's proceedings. The adjudicators are mostly university students who had participated in such events as school students. For some of the teachers and adjudicators, the evening provides the opportunity to catch up after long absences. There is certainly a feeling of community amongst the elite.

There are several tiers of debaters with the largest investment placed in the most senior students. The competition is intense and Leafy Suburbs College encourages older students to mentor younger teams. Some of the Leafy Suburbs College teams congregate without a teacher to oversee their participation. The talk amongst Leafy Suburbs College students is animated. There is no doubt that for many this competition is about beating the 'snobby' schools and that debating is simply the medium. Daniel describes how he makes a point of wearing his uniform in a dishevelled manner so as to conform to what he describes as 'their' expectation of government school students. He argues this is his ploy to get them off-guard. They underestimate their opponents and thereby lose momentum when they recognise the talent of the dishevelled. In this context, winning has a particular salience. The debate begins and while the Leafy Suburbs College students display passion, creativity, and powerful arguments, they are outperformed by a team from one of Melbourne's most prestigious schools. By comparison, their opponents' performance is well choreographed, well rehearsed, and highly polished. Certainly the Leafy Suburbs College students could not understand why they had lost the debate given the clarity, coherence, and creativity of their arguments and the fact that the adjudicator had attested to this in her scoring of the debate. On close examination of the adjudicator's scoring sheet, they learn that their score had suffered due to poor manner. According to the relevant handbook for scoring debates, manner refers to body language, vocal style, humour, personal attacks on opponents, and dress. The students from Leafy Suburbs College are left to find their own way home and meet with the teacher who coordinates the program during their weekly lunchtime meeting. None of their teachers were present at their debate. Their opponents are led out of the room by their specific debating coach, who suggests they meet immediately and consider their strengths and areas for further improvement.

There are indications that those students from government schools who gain places at elite universities do at least as well, if not better, than those from elite Catholic and independent schools (McKenzie and Schweitzer 2001; Murphy, Papanicolaou, and McDowell 2001; Dobson and Skuja 2005). Perhaps a contributing reason is the powerful lessons in strategic choice making provided by a school such as Leafy Suburbs College. In a school where more has to be done with less, choices can be stark. Here, choice has been considered in relation to student identity as a form of negotiation mediating various student subcultures, the dominant school discourses, and students' imagined futures. A major aim has been to consider students' experiences of a school that is both a burden and a privilege. Their engagement with the formal and informal cultures of the school has been explored in relation to subcultures and their imagined futures. The way students work within and between the various student subcultures and dominant renditions of the 'good student' in order to facilitate identities that are both given and adopted has been discussed.

I am arguing that students are agentic in terms of imagining their futures and understanding the place of schooling in the process whereby these might be achieved. They are also well aware of the dominant culture of the school and the student subcultures that coexist in its fissures. I would like to make the case that students, despite our tendency as teachers, parents, and researchers, to underestimate their capacities, have come to understand schooling as the matrix or screen that blurs the boundaries between the real and the imagined. Zizek's argues that

> what I will become depends on the interplay between contingent social circumstances and my free choice ... The crucial point here is, that in certain specific social conditions (of commodity exchange and a global market economy), 'abstraction' becomes a direct feature of actual social life, the way concrete individuals behave and relate to their fate and to their social surroundings.
>
> (Zizek 2000:105)

It is perhaps possible to argue that in order for a government school to succeed in traditional terms, it needs to offer a very narrow interpretation of academic culture. At such a school, the contingent social forces provide students with harsh lessons in choice making. In their early years of secondary schooling, they are introduced to a range of student subcultures. By the end of Year 10, they need to make choices about which school and subjects best facilitate their imagined futures. Working within and between the subcultures and the dominant cultures of the school is their way of relating their fate to their social surroundings. Zizek identifies ideology as

> a matrix that regulates the relationship between visible and nonvisible. Between imaginable and nonimaginable, as well as the changes in this relationship.
>
> (Zizek 1994:1)

He argues that the capacity to see beyond what is identified as already there is critical to debates about change. These insights offer some way of understanding the experience at Leafy Suburbs College. How much is students' engagement with the school shaped by their capacity to see beyond what is identified — both in terms of the matrix that regulates their everyday experience of schooling and their capacity to imagine futures for themselves? My argument is that student subcultures become a critical mediating space between the imaginable and nonimaginable. Through these subcultures, students move between various ways of being and come to understand how these engage with the matrix of ideology.

Many of us share intuitive feelings that there are ways of being, that in their own right, are constituted as nonpreferred by the system. How do we come to understand why the 'nonpreferred' succeed without forgoing their difference? This is particularly interesting in a climate that increasingly 'uncomplicates' success by judging academic excellence more narrowly and in response develops an increasingly instrumentalist system of schooling. I have argued that the answer may be linked to students' facility with strategic identification. In line with Bauman's (2000) contention that a fixed identity is increasingly a liability, students who can 'synthesise self', are most likely to succeed. Like Sebastian and Julian, they move between identities, forever keeping us guessing. For Sebastian and Julian, this is the opposite to students they describe as 'gangster types' who place a high premium on strident identification. These are students who, in their terms, acquire a 'collective subjectivity'. According to Sebastian and Julian, such students 'band together with those who are like-minded or similarly disadvantaged to kind of make a changing situation'. There is a paradox of belonging described here — those who experience oppression are also most likely to form the 'collective subjectivities' that are least suited to 'liquid modernity' (Bauman 2000). If Leafy Suburbs College is anything to go by, there is some evidence that supports the relationship between strident identification and lack of academic success.

Bibliography

Alvesson, M. & Skoloberg, K. (2000), *Reflexive Methodology: New vistas for qualitative research*, London: Sage.
Anderson, B. (2003), *Imagined Communities – Reflections on the origin and spread of nationalism*, London: Verso.
Archer, L. & Francis, B. (2005), 'They never go off the rails like other ethnic groups: teachers' constructions of British Chinese pupils' gender identities and approaches to learning', *British Journal of Sociology of Education*, 26 (2), 165–82.
Australian Bureau of Statistics (ABS) (2004), *Schools Bulletin*, 4221.0, Canberra.
Ball, S. (2003), 'The risks of social reproduction: The middle class and education markets', *London Review of Education,* 1 (3), 163–75.
—— Davies, J., David, M. & Reay, D. (2002), ' "Classification" and "judgement": social class and the "cognitive structures" of choice of higher education', *British Journal of Sociology of Education*, 23 (1), 51–72.
Bauman, Z. (1997), *Postmodernity and its Discontents*, New York: New York University Press.
—— (2000), *Liquid Modernity*, Cambridge, UK: Polity Press.
—— (2004), *Identity*, Cambridge, UK: Polity Press.
Beauchamp, P. (2005), 'Free education costs us $5m', *Herald Sun*, 10 October.
Belfield, C. & Levin, H. (2002), 'The effects of competition between schools on educational outcomes: a review for the United States', *Review of Educational Research*, 72 (2), 279–341.
Benhabib, S. (1995), 'Feminism and postmodernism', in S. Benhabib, J. Butler, D. Cornell, and N. Fraser, *Feminist Contentions – A philosophical exchange*, New York: Routledge.
Bennett, S. E. (2003), 'Coeducation: a risky venture still?', Proceedings of the AARE Annual Conference Auckland, December.

Benvenuto, B. & Kennedy, R. (1986), *Works of Jacques Lacan: An introduction*, London: Free Association Press.
Birrell, B. & Khoo, S. E. (1995), *The Second Generation in Australia: Educational and occupational characteristics*, Bureau of Immigration, Multicultural and Population Research, Canberra: Australian Government Publishing Service (AGPS).
Birrell, B., Rapson, V., Dobson, I. R. & Smith, T. F. (2002), *From Place to Place: School, location and access to university education in Victoria*, Centre for Population and Urban Research, Melbourne: Monash University.
Birrell, B. & Seitz, A. (1986), 'The Mty of ethnic inequality in Australian education', *Journal of the Australian Population Association*, 3 (1), 52–74.
Bottomley, G. (1979), *After the Odyssey: A study of Greek Australians*, St Lucia: University of Queensland Press.
—— (1992), *From Another Place: Migration and the politics of culture*, London and Melbourne: Cambridge University Press.
Bourdieu, P. (1977), *Outline of a Theory of Practice*, London: Cambridge University Press.
—— (1988), *Homo Academicus*, Cambridge, UK Polity Press/Basil Blackwell.
Bradley, S., Draco, M. and Green, C. (2004), 'School Performance in Australia: Is There a Role for Quasi Markets?', *Australian Economic Review*, 37 (3), 271–86.
Britzman, D. (1995), ' "The question of belief"; writing poststructural ethnography', *International Journal of Qualitative Studies in Education*, 8 (39), 252–67.
Burke, G. (2001), 'Funding schools', Paper presented to the National Summit on School Education, Melbourne, 28 September.
Burke, G. & Spaull, A. (2001), 'Australian schools: participation and funding 1901 to 2000', in *2001 Year Book Australia*, Canberra: Australian Bureau of Statistics, 433–46, Australian Bureau of Statistics website.
Butler, J. (1999), 'Performativity's social magic', in J. Butler, *Bourdieu: A critical reader*, London: Blackwell.
Calderon, A., Dobson I. R. & Wentworth, N. (2000), 'Recipe for success: Year 12 subject choice and the transition from school to university', *Journal of Institutional Research*, 9 (1), 111–23.
Caldwell, B. & Roskam, J. (2002), *Australia's Education Choices – A report to the Menzies Research Centre*, Canberra: Menzies Research Centre.
Castles, S., Cope, B., Kalantzis, M. & Morrissey, M. (1988), *Mistaken Identity: Multiculturalism and the demise of nationalism in Australia*, Sydney: Pluto Press.
Clifford, J. (1986), 'Introduction: partial truths', in J. Clifford and G. Marcus (eds), *Writing culture: the poetics and politics of ethnography*, Berkeley: Univerisity of California Press.
Collins, C., Kenway, J. & McLeod, J. (2000), *Factors influencing the educational performance of males and females in school and their initial destinations after leaving school*, Canberra: Department of Education, Training and Youth Affairs (DETYA).
Commonwealth of Australia (1998), *A class act*, Canberra: Senate Employment, Education and Training References.
Connell, R. W. (2004), 'Working-class parents' views of secondary education', *International Journal of Inclusive Education*, 8 (3), 227–239.
DeKoven, M. (2004), *Utopia limited – The sixties and the emergence of the postmodern*, Durham, and London: Duke University Press.
Denzin, N. & Lincoln, Y., (eds) (2000), *Handbook of qualitative research*, Thousand Oaks, CA, and London: Sage.
Dobson, I. & Skuja, E. (2005), 'Secondary schooling, tertiary entry ranks and university

performance', *People and Place*, 13 (1), Melbourne: Centre for Population and Urban Research, Monash University.
Eagleton, T. (2000), *The Idea of Culture*, Oxford: Blackwell.
Edwards, D., Birrell, B. & Smith, T. F. (2005), *Unequal Access to University Places*, Melbourne: Centre for Population and Urban Research, Monash University.
Fuchs, S. (2001), *Against Essentialism – A theory of culture and society*, Cambridge, MA.: Harvard University Press.
Fuery, P. & Mansfield, N. (1997), *Cultural Studies and the New Humanities: Concepts and controversies*, Melbourne: Oxford University Press.
Fullerton, S. (2002), 'Student engagement with school: individual and school-level influences', in *Longitudinal Surveys of Australian Youth*, Research Report Number 27, Melbourne: Australian Council for Education Research (ACER).
Gannicott, K. (1998), ' "League tables" of school performance – A legitimate tool of public policy, *Policy*, Spring, 17–22.
Giddens, A. (1991), *Modernity and Self-identity: Self and society in the late modern age*, Palo Alto, CA: Stanford University Press.
Green, S. (2005), 'Lessons on struggle street', *Education News*, from <www.theage.com.au>, 28 March.
Grosz, E. (1988), 'Desire, the body and recent French feminisms', *Intervention*, 21/22, 28–33.
—— (1990), *Jacques Lacan: A feminist introduction*, Sydney: Allen & Unwin.
Hage, G. (1998), *White Nation: Fantasies of white supremacy in a multicultural society*, Sydney: Pluto Press.
—— (2003), *Against Paranoid Nationalism: Searching for hope in a shrinking society*, Sydney: Pluto Press.
Hawkes, D. (2003), *Ideology*, London and New York: Routledge.
Kenway, J. & Willis, S. (1986), 'Feminist single-sex educational strategies: some theoretical flaws and practical fallacies', *Discourse: Studies in the Cultural Politics of Education*, 7 (1), 1–30.
Ketchell, M. (2001), 'Parents billed for voluntary fees', *Age*, 17 October, p. 5.
Khoo, S. E., McDonald, P., Giorgas, D. & Birrell, B. (2002), *Second Generation Australians*, Canberra: Department of Immigration, Multiculturalism and Indigenous Affairs (DIMIA), retrieved from <www.immi.gov.au>.
Kift, T. (2004), 'Parents zoom in on schools zones, push up prices', *Age*, Domain, 10 October, p. 3.
Kosky, L. (2002), *Improved Educational Outcomes: A better reporting and accountability system for schools*, Melbourne, Victorian Government Department of Education and Training.
Lacan, J. 'The mirror stage as formative of the function of the I as revealed in psychoanalytic experience delivered at the 16th International Congress of Pshychoanalysis, Zürich, 17 July 1949', in *Écrits: a selection / Jacques Lacan* (1997), London: Tavistock.
Lingard, B., Knight J. & Porter P. (eds) (1993), *Schooling reform in hard times*, London: Falmer Press.
Lucey, H. & Reay, D. (2002), 'A market in waste: psychic and structural dimensions of school-choice policy in the UK and children's narratives on "demonized" schools', *Discourse: Studies in the Cultural Politics of Education*, 23 (3), 253–66.
Macguire, M., Ball, S. & McCrae, S. (2001), 'In all our interests': internal marketing at Northwark Park School', *British Journal of the Sociology of Education*, 22 (1), 35–49.
Marginson, S. (1997), *Markets in Education*, Sydney: Allen & Unwin.
Martino, W. & Pallotta-Chiarolli, M. (2001), *Boys' Stuff: Boys talking about what matters*, Sydney: Allen & Unwin.
—— (2003), *So What's a Boy?: Addressing issues of masculinity and schooling*, Berkshire: Open University Press.

McGaw, B., Banks, D. & Piper, K. (1991), *Effective Schools: Schools that make a difference*, Melbourne: ACER.

McKenzie, K. & Schweitzer, R. (2001), 'Who succeeds at university? Factors predicting academic performance in first year Australian university students', *Higher Education Research and Development*, 20 (1), 21–33.

Milligan, S. (1994), *Women in the Teaching Profession*, Canberra: AGPS.

Murphy, M., Papanicolaou, K. & McDowell, R. (2001), 'Entrance score and performance: a three year study of success', *Journal of Institutional Research*, 10 (2), 32–49.

Naylor, R. & Smith, J. (2002), 'Schooling effects on subsequent university performance: evidence for the UK university population', *Warwick Economic Research Papers*, No. 657, Warwick: Department of Economics, University of Warwick.

Neuman, W. L. (2003), *Social Research Methods Qualitative and Quantitative Approaches*, Boston: Allyn & Bacon.

Nieto, S. (2005), 'Public eduction in the twentieth century and beyond: high hopes, broken promises, and an uncertain future', *Harvard Educational Review*, Spring, 75, 43–61.

O'Brien, L. M. & Schillaci, M. (2002), Why do I want to teach, anyway? Utilising autobiography in teacher education, *Teaching Education*, 13 (1), 25–40.

Pollock, D. (ed.) (1997), *Exceptional Spaces: Essays in performance and history*, Chapel Hill: University of North Carolina Press.

Pope, D. (2001), *'Doing School': How we are creating a generation of stressed out, materialistic, and miseducated students*, New Haven, CT and London: Yale University Press.

Portes, A. & Rumbaut, R. (2001), *Legacies, the Story of the Immigrant Second Generation*, Berkeley: University of California Press.

Poynting, S. (2002), 'Bin Laden in the suburbs: attacks on Arab and Muslim Australians before and after 11 September', *Current Issues in Criminal Justice*, 14 (1), 43–64.

Rapoport, T. & Lomsky-Feder, E. (2002), ' "Intelligentsia" as an ethnic habitus: the inculcation and restructuring of intelligenstia among Russian Jews', *British Journal of Sociology of Education*, 23 (2), 233–48.

Rindfleisch, T. (2002), 'Fee tactics rile parents', *Sunday Herald Sun*, 3 February, p. 16.

Rowe, K. J. (2000), 'Assessment, league table and school effectiveness: consider the facts and "let's gets real"!', *Journal of Educational Enquiry*, 1 (1), 72–99.

Sarup, M. (1992), *Jacques Lacan*, Hertfordshire: Harvester Wheatsheaf.

Sartre, J.-P. (2004), *The Imaginary – A phenomenological psychology of the imagination*, London and New York: Routledge.

Saukko, P. (2003), *Doing Research in Cultural Studies*, London and Thousand Oaks, CA: Sage.

Skeggs, B. (2004), *Class, Self, Culture*, London: Routledge.

Smith, D. (1987), *The Everyday World as Problematic: A feminist sociology*, Milton Keynes, UK and New York: Open University Press.

Spivak, G. (1993) *Outside in the Teaching Machine*, New York and London: Routledge.

Steinberg, J. (2002), *The Gatekeepers: Inside the admissions process of a premier college*, New York: Viking.

Stronach, I. & MacLure, M. (1997), *Educational research undone: the postmodern embrace*, Buckingham, UK: Open University Press.

Teese., R. (2000), *Academic Success and Social Power – Examinations and inequality*, Melbourne: Melbourne University Press.

Teese, R. & Polesel, J. (2003), *Undemocratic Schooling – Equity and quality in mass secondary education in Australia*, Melbourne: Melbourne University Press.

Tomazin, F. (2004), 'The new class struggle is about getting into school', *Age*, 7 June, p. 6.

Tsolidis, G. (1986), *Educating Voula – A report on non-English-speaking background girls and education*, Melbourne: Victorian Government Ministry of Education.

—— (1995), 'Greek-Australian Families', in R. Hartley (ed.), *Families and Cultural Diversity*, Sydney: Allen & Unwin and Australian Institute of Family Studies.

—— (2000), 'Diasporic youth: moving beyond the academic versus the popular in school cultures', in J. McLeod & K. Malone (eds), *Researching Youth, Australian*, Hobart: Clearinghouse for Youth Studies.

—— (2001a), 'Diasporic maternity — Australia, Canada and Greece', *Social Semiotics*, 11A, 193–208.

—— (2001b), *Schooling, Diaspora and Gender – Being feminist and being different*, London: Open University Press.

—— (2003), 'Mothers, memories and cultural imaginings', *Greek Review of Social Research Special Issue — Gender and international migration: focus on Greece*, 110A, 141–63.

UNESCO (1998), *Learning: The treasure within*, Paris: UNESCO Publishing and the Australian National Commission for UNESCO.

Van Maanen, J. (1995), *Representation in Ethnography*, Thousand Oak, CA: Sage.

Vasta, E. & S. Castles (eds) (1996), *The Teeth are Smiling: The persistence of racism in multicultural Australia*, Sydney: Allen & Unwin.

Victorian Curriculum and Assessment Authority, State Government of Victoria (2005), <www.vcaa.vic.edu.au/vcal/students/wherewillvcaltakeme.html>.

Vincent, C. (2001), 'Social class and parental agency', *Journal of Education Policy*, 16 (4), 347–64.

Weis, L. & Fine, M. (2000), *Speed Bumps: A student-friendly guide to qualitative research*, New York: Teachers College Press.

—— (2001), 'Extraordinary conversations in public schools', *Qualitative Studies in Education*, 14 (4) 497–523.

Whitty, G., Power, S. & Halpin, D. (1998), *Devolution and Choice in Education: The school, the state and the market*, Melbourne: ACER.

Williams, R. (1980), '*Utopia and science fiction'*, in *Problems in Materialism and Culture: Selected essays*, London: New Left Books, 196–212.

Willis, P. (2003), 'Foot soldiers of modernity: the dialectics of cultural consumption and the 21st century school', *Harvard Educational Review*, 3 (73), 390–415.

Yates, L. (2004), *What Does Good Education Research Look Like?*, Berkshire, UK: Open University Press.

Yates, L. & Leder, G. (1996), *Student Pathways: A review and overview of national databases on gender equity*, Canberra: Department of Education and Training and Children's, Youth and Family Bureau.

Yon, D. (2000), 'Urban portraits of identity: on the problem of knowing culture and identity in intercultural studies', *Journal of Intercultural Studies*, 21 (2), 143–57.

Zizek, S. (2001), *Enjoy Your Symptom! Jacques Lacan in Hollywood and out*, New York and London: Routledge.

—— (2000), 'Class struggle or postmodernism? Yes please!', in J. Butler, E. Laclau and S. Zizek (2000), *Contingency, Hegemony, Universality – Contemporary uialogues on the Left*, London and New York: Verso.

—— (ed.) (1994), *Mapping ideology*, London and New York: Verso.

Index

Alternative College 174–176, 195
Asian 60, 82, 98
Australian 58–60, 98
'blonde' girls 64, 69, 74–76, 89–91
Class
    middle–class 5, 48–50
    working–class 5, 49–50
Culture
    of school 5–8, 111, 121, 141, 147, 156, 159, 173
    of success 33, 146, 147, 179
Enrolments 41, 43–44
Ethnic minority 7, 81
Ethnography 6, 13–15
Gender 64
Greek 91, 98, 102–103
'hardcores' 63
Identity 6–8, 10–11, 57, 131, 147, 197–198
Imagination 27–29
Imagined futures 4, 6, 11, 180, 188–190, 197
'jocks' 56, 58, 60, 63–64, 70, 72, 74–76, 88, 190
Jewish 60, 118–120, 122,
Lacan, J. 28–30
'musos' 61, 108, 113, 117, 122,184, 192
Matrix, The 21–25, 28
Migrants 50, 62
Music 126–127, 136–137

'nerds' 58, 70, 72, 143
'popular' kids 58
Postmodernism 6, 9, 24
Private school 4, 191, 193
Public school 4, 10, 193, 197
Refusal of choice 9–10
Research 12, 68–69, 91
Russians 99–100
School
    discipline 165–166, 168, 182
    fees 5
    results 9, 35–40, 93, 101, 109
    uniform 165–166, 168
    zones 40–44
Schooling 5–8, 23, 192
Sexuality 64
    heterosexuality 74, 86
    homophobia 76
    homosexuality 70
Social justice 6–9, 23–24
Subcultures 6–7, 11, 56, 63–64, 67–69, 109, 125, 128, 140–142, 192, 197–198
University
    entry to 4–8, 52, 141, 1991, 197
Utopia 26–28
'wogs' 59, 65, 83–86, 89–90, 98, 105, 148, 192–94
Zizek, S. 9, 24–25, 28

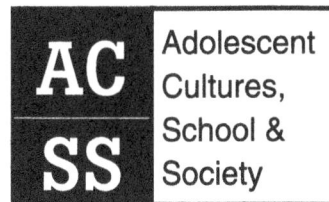

Adolescent Cultures, School & Society

Joseph L. DeVitis & Linda Irwin-DeVitis
GENERAL EDITORS

As schools struggle to redefine and restructure themselves, they need to be cognizant of the new realities of adolescents. Thus, this series of monographs and textbooks is committed to depicting the variety of adolescent cultures that exist in today's post-industrial societies. It is intended to be a primarily qualitative research, practice, and policy series devoted to contextual interpretation and analysis that encompasses a broad range of interdisciplinary critique. In addition, this series will seek to provide a pragmatic, pro-active response to the current backlash of conservatism that continues to dominate political discourse, practice, and policy. This series seeks to address issues of curriculum theory and practice; multicultural education; aggression and violence; the media and arts; school dropouts; homeless and runaway youth; alienated youth; at-risk adolescent populations; family structures and parental involvement; and race, ethnicity, class, and gender studies.

Send proposals and manuscripts to the general editors at:
>Joseph L. DeVitis & Linda Irwin-DeVitis
The John H. Lounsbury School of Education
Georgia College & State University
Campus Box 70
Milledgeville, GA 31061-0490

To order other books in this series, please contact our Customer Service Department at:
>(800) 770-LANG (within the U.S.)
(212) 647-7706 (outside the U.S.)
(212) 647-7707 FAX

or browse online by series at:
>WWW.PETERLANG.COM